RAPID ANALYSIS

OF

ELECTROCARDIOGRAMS

A Self-Study Program

RAPID ANALYSIS

OF

ELECTROCARDIOGRAMS

A SELF-STUDY PROGRAM
Second Edition

**EMANUEL STEIN, M.D., M.P.H.
F.A.C.P., F.A.C.C., F.C.C.P.**

Professor of Internal Medicine and
Professor of Family and Community Medicine
Eastern Virginia Medical School
Norfolk, Virginia
Medical Director, United States Public Health Service, Ret.
Diplomate, American Board of Internal Medicine and
Subspecialty Board of Cardiovascular Disease

Illustrations by
THOMAS XENAKIS, M.A., A.M.I.

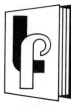

Lea & Febiger   1992   Philadelphia • London

Lea & Febiger
200 Chester Field Parkway
Malvern, Pennsylvania 19355-9725
(215) 251-2230

Executive Editor—R. Kenneth Bussy
Project Editor—Tanya Lazar
Production Manager—Samuel A. Rondinelli

Library of Congress Cataloging-in-Publication Data

Stein, Emanuel.
    Rapid analysis of electrocardiograms (ECGs) : a self-study program /   Emanuel Stein : illustrations
by Thomas Xenakis.—2nd ed.
      p.   cm.
    Rev. ed. of: Clinical electrocardiography. 1987.
    Includes bibliographical references and index.
    ISBN 0-8121-1441-8
    1. Electrocardiography. 2. Heart—Diseases—Diagnosis.
I. Stein, Emanuel. Clinical electrocardiography. II. Title.
    [DNLM: 1. Electrocardiography—problems. WG 18 S819r]
RC683.5.E5S75 1992
616.1'207547—dc20
DNLM/DLC
for Library of Congress   91-33729
                                                     CIP

First Edition, 1987
Reprinted 1987, 1988, 1990, 1991

PRINTED IN THE UNITED STATES OF AMERICA

Print No.   5   4   3   2   1

THIS WORK IS LOVINGLY DEDICATED

TO MY WIFE AND CHILDREN

for their great love, abundant
support, patience and understanding

TO MY TEACHERS

who spanned the entire experience of
electrocardiography

TO MY STUDENTS

in the classroom and in the clinic,
from whom I continue to learn

TO MY FUTURE STUDENTS

who will benefit from this effort

Preface

This book is simply written and amply illustrated to provide a firm foundation in electrocardiography for all interested members of the health professions. Some may rightfully feel that a particular subject should have been included or given more weight and that other areas have been emphasized too much. I accept full responsibility for the allocation of priorities in this synthesis of vast amounts of material. The electrocardiograms have been chosen with great care and confirmed, where possible, by clinical-pathological correlation, cardiac catheterization, X-ray and noninvasive techniques. When the question arose as to absolute accuracy versus ease of understanding in a given illustration, the decision generally was made in favor of ease of understanding. Following the adage that a picture is worth a thousand words, each illustration is carefully coordinated with the short text below it. Self-assessment is emphasized in this self-learning, programmed course, with questions on most pages, based on the text and reflected in the illustrations. The notes and reference section at the end of the book comprise additional topics, important to the understanding of heart rhythms, including: ladder diagrams, reentry and enhanced automaticity, concealed conduction, "rule of bigeminy," fusion (including Dressler beats), parasystole, aberrant ventricular conduction (including the Ashman phenomenon), His bundle studies, the Lown-Ganong-Levine syndrome, rate dependent left bundle branch block, sinoatrial Wenckebach periods, and atrioventricular block versus atrioventricular dissociation. Because a step-by-step approach is followed, it is advisable to start at the beginning and progress systematically through the book. After you have learned the basic principles of electrocardiography and have completed all the exercises and practice electrocardiograms, the book can serve as a study guide as well as a teaching, reference, and review manual. As a review, the basic principles of electrocardiography can be covered in one sitting. This method of learning to interpret electrocardiograms has been received with excitement and enthusiasm in the classroom and in the clinic.

The book is divided into six chapters. The first chapter introduces the basic concepts of electrocardiography, using the vector approach.[1-3] The characteristics of the normal electrocardiogram are explained and illustrated. The normal 12-lead electrocardiogram is then completely analyzed. Discussions of abnormal states, including hypertrophy, ventricular repolarization alterations, myocardial infarction, conduction disturbances, and arrhythmias, comprise the remaining five chapters.

At the end of each chapter are several practice electrocardiograms related to that chapter. The analysis follows each practice electrocardiogram. Fifty additional electrocardiograms are then presented, relating to all the chapters for practice and review. In this era of high technology, most of the electrocardiograms in this section have been recorded on the multichannel system in common use in most hospitals. These electrocardiograms are mounted to preserve the simultaneous recording of the various leads. They have been altered only to fit the page. Here too, the analysis follows each practice electrocardiogram. It is hoped that this introduction will stimulate you to continue learning and reading electrocardiograms.

I have had the opportunity of reaching thousands of people during my decades in medical practice and tens of thousands more through my books and courses. If I have made life and learning easier I shall treasure it as a major accomplishment of my lifetime.

I thank Mr. R. Kenneth Bussy and Mr. Samuel Rondinelli of Lea & Febiger for their help in making this book possible and Mr. Thomas Xenakis for elegantly translating my drawings. I add my appreciation to Dr. William Fox,[4] Dr. David B. Propert, and Dr. Donald W. Drew for providing electrocardiograms that have enriched this work.

Norfolk, Virginia   Emanuel Stein, M.D.

> All references are found on pages 397 to 400.

Contents

Chapter *1*

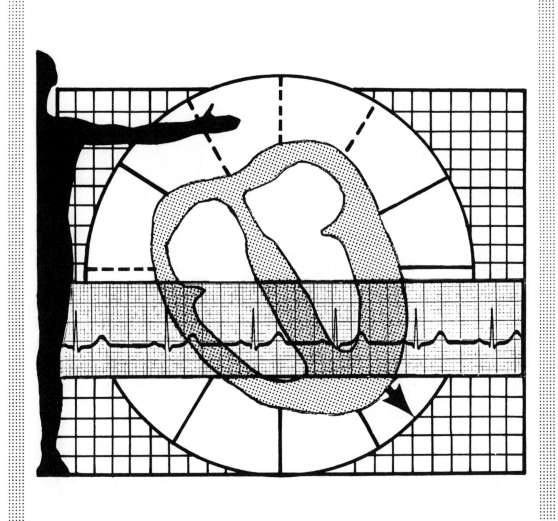

Basic Concepts and The Normal
Electrocardiogram

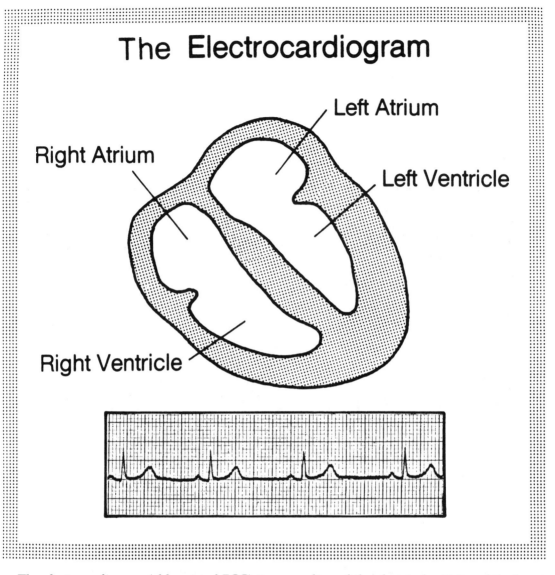

The electrocardiogram (abbreviated ECG) is a recording of the electrical activity of the heart from the body surface. By the placement of electrodes on designated areas of the body, we usually record 12 views of this electrical activity. All four chambers, the left and right atria and the left and right ventricles, are represented on this recording.

The electrocardiogram (ECG) is a recording of the _____   electrical
activity of the heart.

The standard electrocardiogram is a recording of _____ views of this   12
electrical activity.

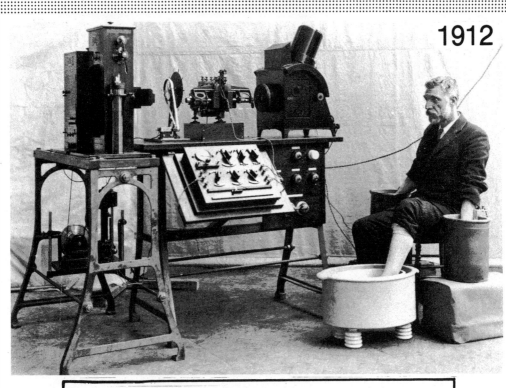

1912

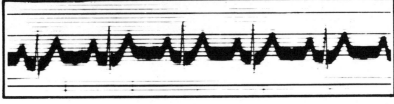

Early Electrocardiogram

It wasn't always easy to take electrocardiograms in the early days of electrocardiography. The patient had to have both arms and the left leg in containers of conducting solution (saline). The electrodes were attached to the containers, not directly to the patient. The large machine stands in sharp contrast to the compact models of today. Willem Einthoven, who contributed greatly to early electrocardiography, is often called the father of electrocardiography.

In the early days of electrocardiography, the electrodes were attached to the containers of conducting solution, not directly to the _____ .

patient

_____ _____ is known as the father of electrocardiography.

Willem Einthoven

Depolarization and Repolarization

(+) (+) (+) (+) (+) (+) (+) (+) (+) (+) (+) (+) (+) (+) (+)
(-) (-) (-) (-) (-) (-) (-) (-) (-) (-) (-) (-) (-) (-) (-)

Cardiac Cell

(-) (-) (-) (-) (-) (-) (-) (-) (-) (-) (-) (-) (-) (-) (-)
(+) (+) (+) (+) (+) (+) (+) (+) (+) (+) (+) (+) (+) (+) (+)

1. Resting or Polarized State

(-) (-) (-) (-) (-) (-) (-) (-) (-) (-) (-) (-) (-) (+) (+) (+) (+)
(+) (+) (+) (+) (+) (+) (+) (+) (+) (+) (+) (-) (-) (-) (-)

(+) (+) (+) (+) (+) (+) (+) (+) (+) (+) (+) (-) (-) (-) (-)
(-) (-) (-) (-) (-) (-) (-) (-) (-) (-) (-) (+) (+) (+) (+)

2. Depolarization, Almost Complete

(-) (-) (-) (+) (+) (+) (+) (+) (+) (+) (+) (+) (+) (+) (+)
(+) (+) (+) (-) (-) (-) (-) (-) (-) (-) (-) (-) (-) (-) (-)

(+) (+) (+) (-) (-) (-) (-) (-) (-) (-) (-) (-) (-) (-) (-)
(-) (-) (-) (+) (+) (+) (+) (+) (+) (+) (+) (+) (+) (+) (+)

3. Repolarization, Almost Complete

The function of the heart is to pump blood for the body's needs. The *mechanical* act of pumping blood is preceded by, and responsive to, an *electrical* stimulus. The electrocardiogram is a recording of these electrical events. In order for current to flow, there must be *positive* $(+)$ and *negative* $(-)$ charges. These are contained in and around the specialized cells of the heart. In the resting state the outside of the cell is more positive relative to the inside of the cell. This is the balanced or *polarized* state, with no flow of electricity. When the polarized cell is stimulated, the polarity

The contraction of the heart is preceded by a(an) _____   electrical
stimulus (or impulse).

In the resting (polarized) state, the outside of the cell is more _____   positive
relative to the inside of the cell.

Physiologic Properties of Myocardial Cells

Automaticity -
Ability to Initiate an Impulse

Excitability -
Ability to Respond to an Impulse

Conductivity -
Ability to Transmit an Impulse

Contractility -
Ability to Respond with Pumping Action

of the cell is reversed. The inside of the cell becomes more positive relative to the outside. This process is known as *depolarization* and reflects the flow of an electrical current to all cells along the pathways of conduction. The cell then returns to its original resting state by the process called *repolarization.* The physiologic properties of myocardial cells permitting these events to occur and leading to contraction of the heart muscle are listed above.

Four physiologic properties of myocardial cells include:

_____ ,   automaticity
_____ ,   excitability
_____ , and   conductivity
_____ .   contractility

Electrical Conduction System of the Heart

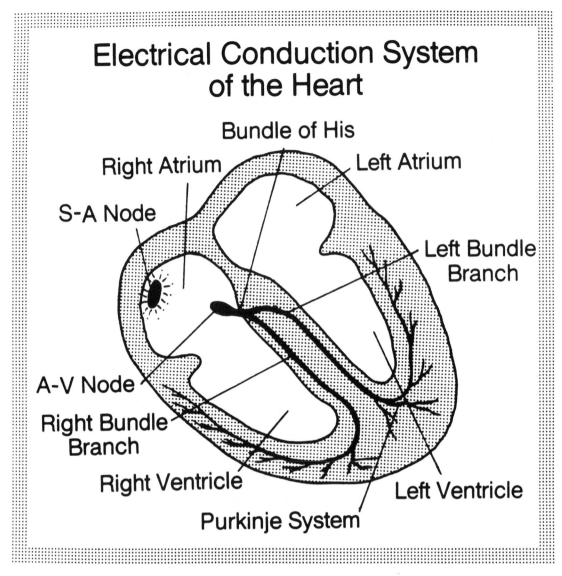

The processes just described follow specific pathways within the heart known as its electrical conduction system. The *sinoatrial (S-A) node* is normally the site of origin of the electrical impulse, leading to depolarization of the atria. The impulse then spreads through the *atrioventricular (A-V) node* and *bundle of His* to the *left (LBB)* and *right (RBB) bundle branches* and then to the ventricles through the *Purkinje fiber network,* leading to ventricular depolarization.

The specific pathways within the heart used by the electrical impulse is known as the _____ _____ _____ .

    electrical conduction system

The normal site of origin of the electrical impulse is the _____ .

    S-A node

Rate of Impulse Formation
(Impulses Per Minute)

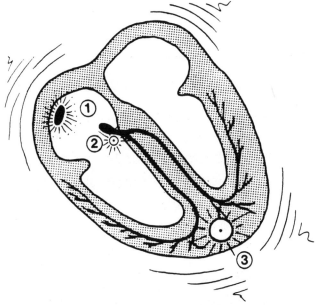

① S-A Node   60-100

② A-V Junction 40-60

③ Ventricle   20-40

Although the primary and dominant pacemaker of the heart is the *S-A node,* under various circumstances and stimuli, another pacemaker may become dominant. There may be two or more pacemakers propagating impulses at the same time. Each pacemaker has its own *inherent rate.* In general, the pacemaker with the fastest inherent rate becomes the dominant cardiac pacemaker. The S-A node emits 60 to 100 impulses per min., the A-V junction 40 to 60 impulses per min. and still lower pacemakers, such as a ventricular pacemaker, 20 to 40 impulses per min. Thus, the S-A node is usually the fastest and dominant cardiac pacemaker. If a secondary pacemaker, such as the junctional or ventricular pacemaker, speeds up, it may become the dominant pacemaker. Also, if the S-A node slows down or fails, a secondary pacemaker may become dominant.

Each pacemaker has its own _____ _____ .   inherent rate

The pacemaker with the fastest inherent rate is usually
the _____ pacemaker.   dominant

Autonomic Nervous System Sympathetic and Parasympathetic Nerves

Sympathetic System
- Supplying both Atria and Ventricles

Mediator - Norepinephrine
Increases:
Rate of S-A Node
Rate of Atrioventricular Conduction
Excitability
Force of Contraction

Parasympathetic System (Vagus Nerve)
- Supplying Atria Primarily

Mediator - Acetylcholine
Decreases:
Rate of S-A Node
Rate of Atrioventricular Conduction
Excitability

The heart is also influenced by both branches of the autonomic nervous system, the *sympathetic* and *parasympathetic nerves*. Stimulation of the sympathetic system, supplying both atria and ventricles, with norepinephrine as the mediator, leads to increased rate of the S-A node, increased atrioventricular conduction, increased excitability and increased force of contraction. Stimulation of the parasympathetic system (vagus nerve), supplying primarily the atria, with acetylcholine as the mediator, leads to decreased rate of the S-A node, decreased atrioventricular conduction, and decreased excitability. If one system is blocked, the effects of the other are seen. For example, if the sympathetic system were blocked, the effects of the parasympathetic system would be elicited.

The sympathetic system with _____ as the mediator affects the _____ and _____ .

    epinephrine
    atria
    ventricles

The parasympathetic system with _____ as the mediator primarily affects the _____ .

    acetylcholine
    atria

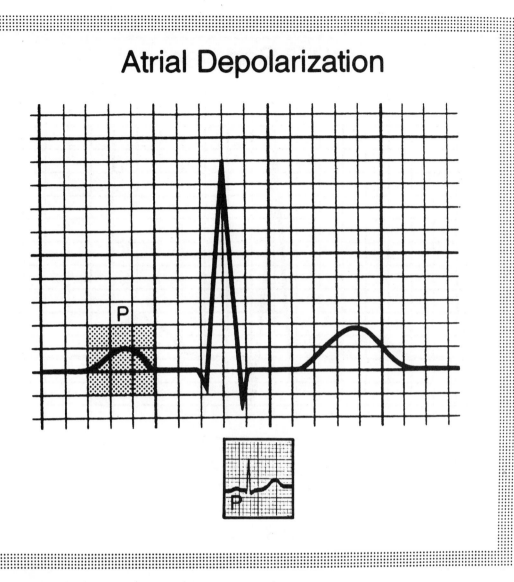

Atrial Depolarization

The wave of depolarization that begins in the S-A node spreads to both atria, first to the right atrium, then to the left atrium. The depolarization of both atria is represented by the *P wave* on the electrocardiogram. The P wave is normally the first electrocardiographic deflection of each cardiac cycle.

The first electrocardiographic deflection of the cardiac cycle is normally the _____ wave.   P

The P wave represents the depolarization of both _____.   atria

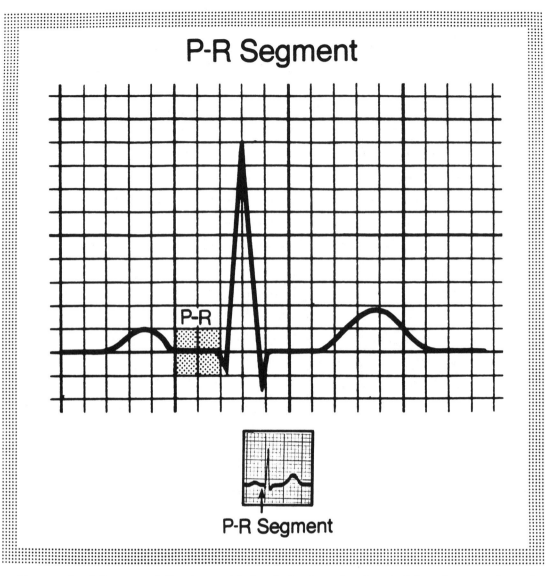

P-R Segment

P-R

P-R Segment

During the *P-R segment,* following atrial depolarization, the electrical impulse spreads to the A-V node, bundle of His, and bundle branches. In the specialized electrophysiology laboratory, recordings can be made from the bundle of His using special recording techniques. On the clinical electrocardiogram, only the flat line is generally seen.

The spread of the electrical impulse through the A-V node, bundle of His, and bundle branches occurs electrocardiographically during the __ _____ .

P-R segment

The P-R segment is usually a _____ _____ on the electrocardiogram.

flat line

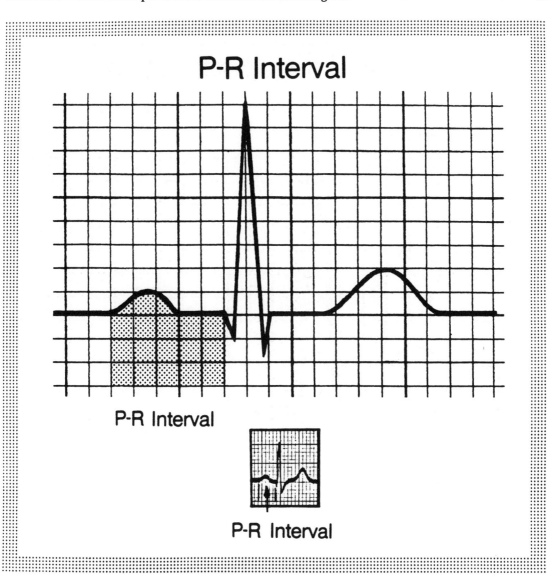

The *P-R interval* includes the P wave and P-R segment. This interval represents the time of transmission of the electrical impulse from the atria to the ventricles.

The _____ _____ represents the time of transmission of the   P-R interval
electrical impulse from the beginning of atrial depolarization to the
beginning of ventricular depolarization.

The P-R interval includes the _____ _____ and   P wave
the _____ _____ .   P-R segment

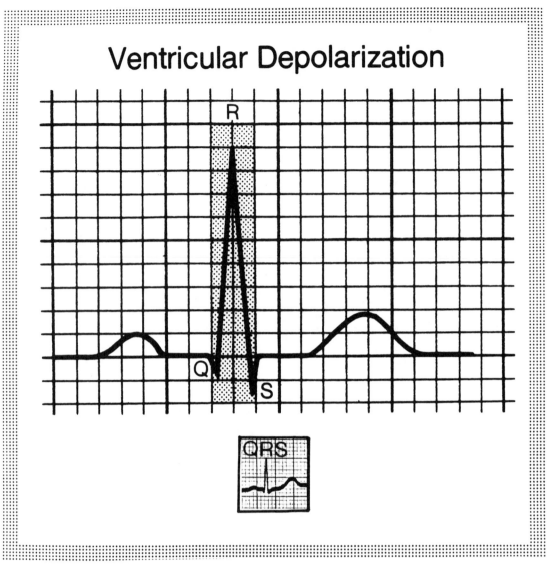

Depolarization of both ventricles is reflected in the *QRS complex*. The *R wave* is the initial positive deflection (upward, above the resting baseline of the electrocardiogram) of the QRS complex. The negative deflection (downward, inverted, occurring below the resting baseline of the electrocardiogram) *before* the R wave is the *Q wave*. The negative deflection *after* the R wave is the *S wave*, which is usually the terminal part of the QRS complex.

**The initial negative deflection, if present, of the QRS complex is
the ___ _____**   Q wave

**The first positive deflection of the QRS complex, whether or not it is
preceded by a negative deflection, is the _____ _____ .**   R wave

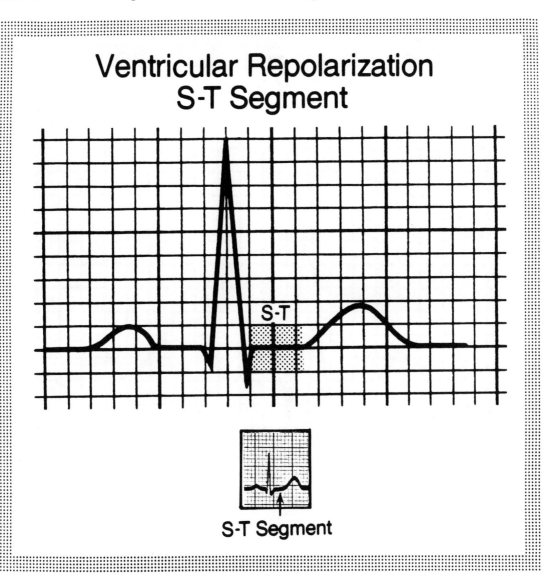

Ventricular Repolarization
S-T Segment

S-T Segment

The *S-T segment* extends from the end of the QRS complex to the beginning of the T wave (see next page). It represents the earlier phase of repolarization of both ventricles. The S-T segment is normally isoelectric (at the same level as the resting baseline). It is neither elevated (positive) nor depressed (negative). The point at which the S-T segment joins the QRS complex is known as the J (junction) point.

The S-T segment is normally _____ .   isolectric

The point at which the S-T segment joins the QRS complex is the ____ _____.   J point

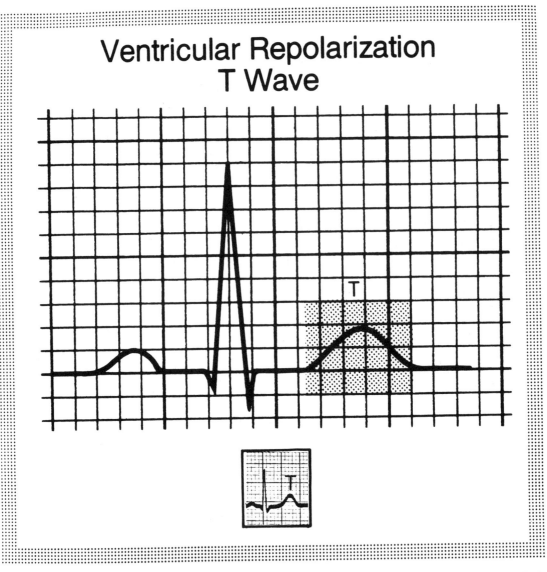

Later repolarization of both ventricles inscribes the *T wave* on the electrocardiogram. The S-T segment and the T wave are sensitive indicators of the status of the ventricular myocardium. *Atrial repolarization* is not often seen on the electrocardiogram because of its small size and because it coincides with the QRS complex.

Ventricular repolarization is represented electrocardiographically by the _____ _____ and the _____ _____.	S-T segment T wave
Atrial repolarization usually is _____ _____ on the electrocardiogram.	not seen

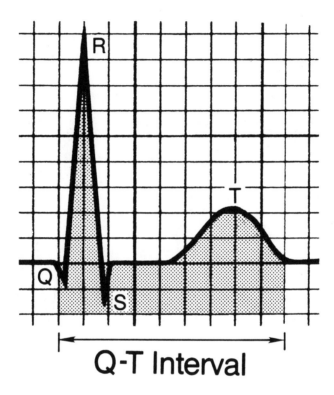

Ventricular
Depolarization and Repolarization
Q-T Interval

Q-T Interval

The Q-T interval includes the QRS complex, S-T segment, and T wave.

The Q-T interval:
extends from the beginning of the _____ wave to   Q
the end of the _____ wave.   T

represents ventricular _____   depolarization
and _____ .   repolarization

Types of Ventricular Complexes (QRS)*

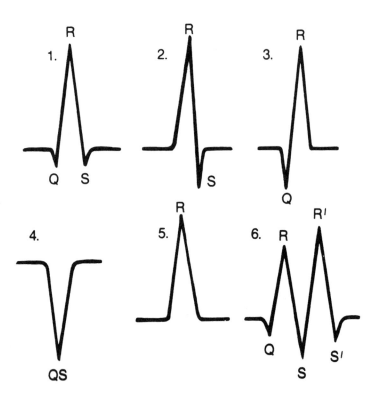

1. QRS; Q wave—negative deflection before the R wave
        R wave—positive deflection
        S wave—negative deflection after the R wave
2. RS; no Q wave present
3. QR; no S wave present
4. QS; totally negative complex, no R wave present
5. R; no Q or S waves present
6. QRSR'S', a second positive deflection after an S wave is an R' (R prime), which, in turn, may be followed by a second negative deflection, an S' (S prime)

The ventricular complexes may also be described using upper and lower case letters indicating the large or small sizes of the waves. For example, the complex in No. 1 may be described as QRS or qRs because the q and s waves are small relative to the R wave. Similarly, No. 2 may be described as RS or Rs, etc. The use of upper and lower case is especially helpful in a written description not accompanied by the actual electrocardiogram.

---

*Although not all the ventricular complexes contain Q, R, and S waves, they are still commonly called QRS complexes.

Practice

Identify the Principal Electrocardiographic Waves (P, QRS and T)

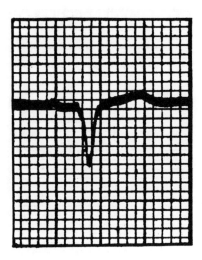

Answer:

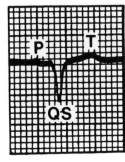

Remember:

The Q wave is ALWAYS negative

The R wave is ALWAYS positive

The S wave is ALWAYS negative

The P and T waves may be positive or negative. When there is no R wave, only one large negative wave, it is called a QS wave, as above.

Practice

Identify the Principal Electrocardiographic Waves (P, QRS and T)

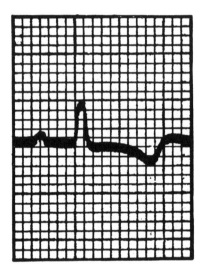

Answer:

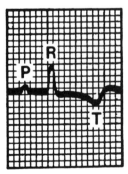

Note again: Although not all the ventricular complexes contain Q, R, and S waves, they are commonly called QRS complexes. Here, the P wave is positive and the T wave is negative.

Practice

Identify the Principal Electrocardiographic Waves (P, QRS and T)

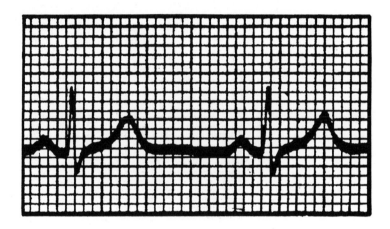

Answer:

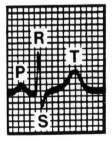

This ventricular complex contains an R wave (positive) and an S wave (negative). Using upper and lower case letters, as explained on page 16, the ventricular complex may be labeled Rs.

Practice

Identify the Principal Electrocardiographic Waves (P, QRS and T)

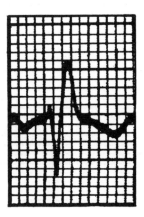

Answer:

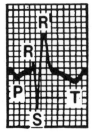

This ventricular complex begins with a small positive deflection, the R wave, followed by a negative deflection, the S wave, then another positive deflection, the R' wave. Both the P and T waves are negative in this lead. Using upper and lower case letters, the ventricular complex may be labeled rSR'.

Practice

Identify the Principal Electrocardiographic Waves (P, QRS and T)

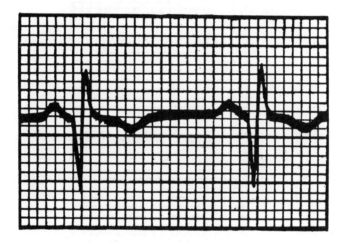

Answer:

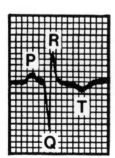

The ventricular complex is initiated by a negative deflection, the Q wave, followed by an R wave. The T wave is negative.

Practice

Identify the Principal Electrocardiographic Waves (P, QRS and T)

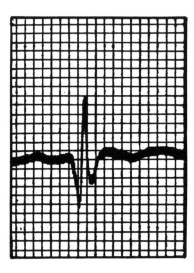

Answer:

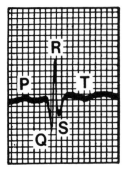

The three components of the QRS complex are seen here—the Q, R, and S waves.

Practice
Label the Electrocardiographic Waves, Intervals and Segments

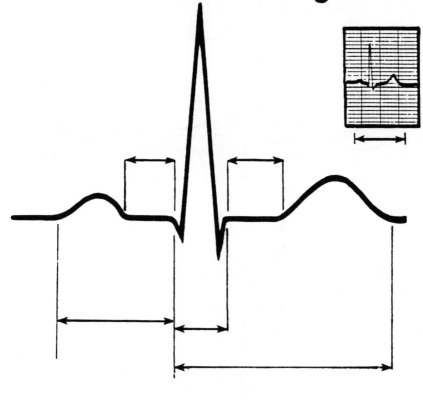

Answer:

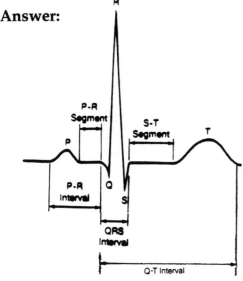

Thorough familiarity with the nomenclature of the components of the cardiac cycle is vital in electrocardiography. Prior to studying the placement of the leads, heart rate determination, and measurements, review all the material studied so far.

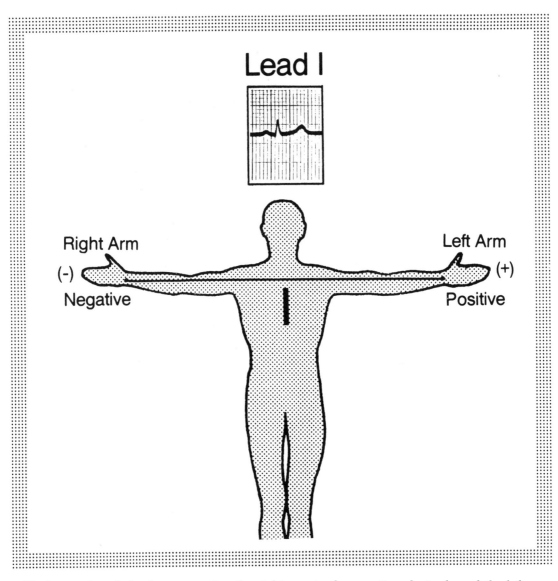

Einthoven found that by connecting the right arm to the negative electrode and the left arm to the positive electrode and inducing a current to flow, certain deflections were recorded, known as *lead I.* For recording, Einthoven used the string galvanometer, a movable writing element within a magnetic field.

The right (−) and left (+) arms comprise lead _____ . I

For recording, Einthoven used
the _____ _____ , a movable writing string galvanometer
element in a magnetic field.

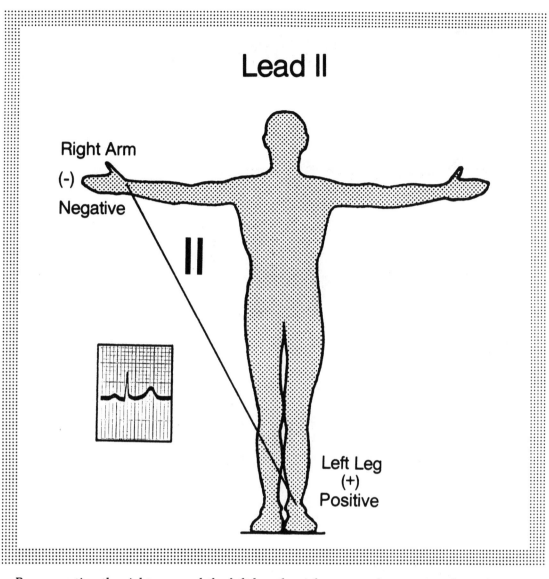

By connecting the right arm and the left leg, the right arm to the negative electrode and the left leg to the positive electrode, Einthoven recorded what became known as *lead II*.

Lead II connects the _____ _____ with   right arm
the _____ _____ .   left leg

The right arm is _____ and the left leg is _____ in lead II.   negative
                                                                           positive

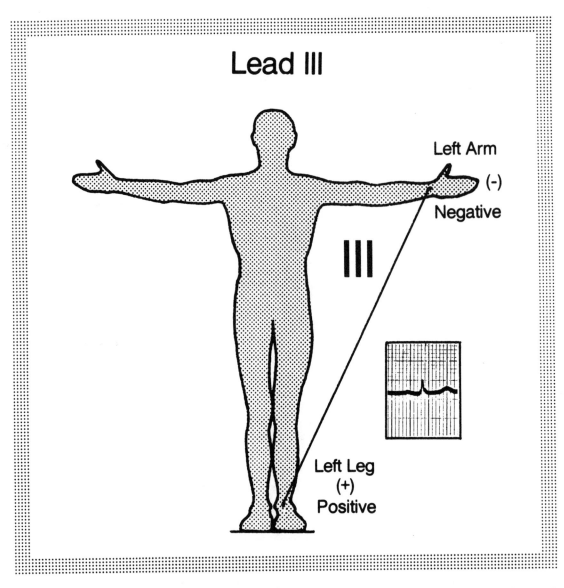

Lead III

By connecting the left arm and the left leg, the left arm to the negative electrode and the left leg to the positive electrode, *lead III* is formed.

Lead III connects the _____ _____ with the _____ _____ .

The left arm is _____ and the left leg is _____ in lead III.

left arm
left leg

negative
positive

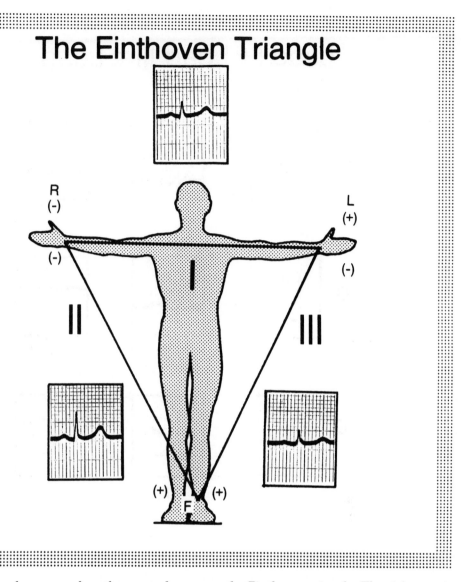

The Einthoven Triangle

These three leads, arranged as above, are known as the Einthoven triangle. The right arm is always *negative* and the left leg is always *positive*. Note the following special relationship:

lead I + lead III = lead II

This is an electrical truth that always holds for the *area* encompassed by each deflection. We use the heights and depths of the deflections as a good approximation. This relationship is further illustrated on the next page.

The Einthoven triangle is composed of leads ____ , ____ , and ____ .   I II III

The summation of the three leads is as follows: leads _____ + _____   I III
= _____ .   II

Lead I + Lead III = Lead II

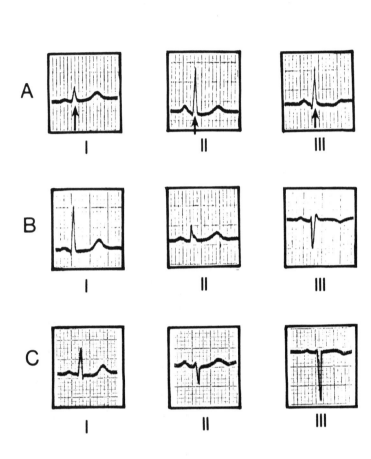

The arrows in A point to the QRS complexes in leads I, II, and III. The deflection in lead I is approximately 3 mm. tall and the deflection in lead III is 9 mm. tall. Using the rule that

$$\text{leads I} + \text{III} = \text{lead II}$$

the lead II deflection must be 12 mm. tall. This is true for the P as well as the T waves. Apply this relationship to B and C above.

The electrical truth, leads I + III = II, always holds for the _____ encompassed by each deflection.   area

As a good approximation of this electrical truth, we use the _____ and _____ of the deflections.   heights depths

Practice

Label the Einthoven triangle, including the polarity (+ or -) of the leads.

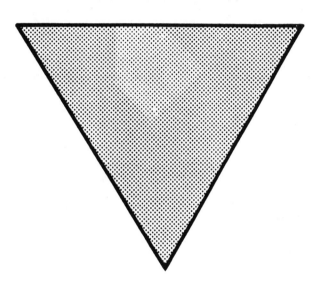

Answer:

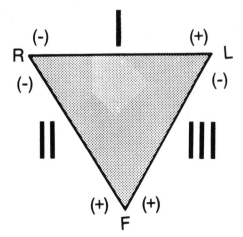

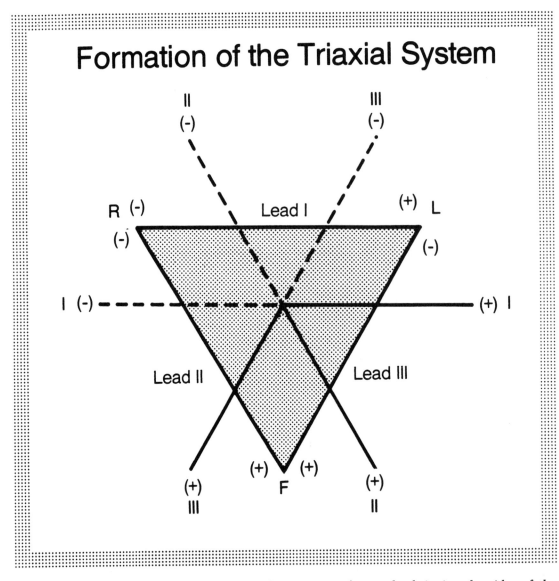

Formation of the Triaxial System

The Einthoven triangle may be converted into a *triaxial system* by bringing the sides of the triangle to the common center. The positives and negatives are now clearly delineated. The solid lines represent the positive half of each lead, whereas the broken lines represent the negative half.

By bringing the sides of the triangle to the common center, the Einthoven triangle may be converted into a _____ system.   triaxial

The triaxial system clearly delineates the _____   positives
and _____ .   negatives

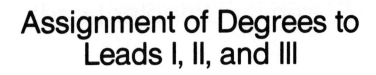

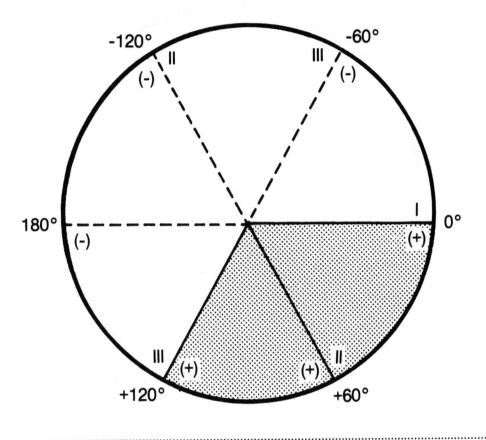

In assigning degrees to the triaxial reference system, the axes are 60° apart. The positions of the positives and negatives remain as in the Einthoven triangle.

Up to now we have been studying three leads, I, II, and III. These are the *bipolar* extremity leads; each lead makes use of two extremities. For many years these were the only leads used in electrocardiography.

Lead I (+) is at _____°.   0
Lead II (+) is at _____°.   +60
Lead III (+) is at _____°.   +120

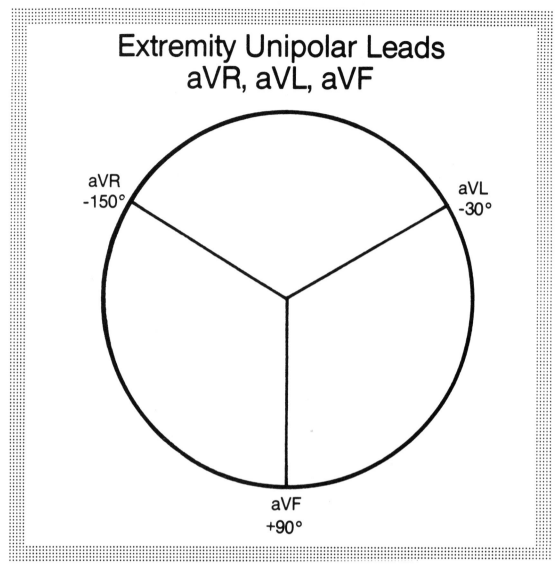

In time, other leads were added, the *unipolar* extremity leads: *aVR (right arm)*, *aVL (left arm)*, and *aVF (left leg)*. Only one pole, the *positive,* is attached to each extremity. The negative is connected to a central terminal. The letter "a" refers to the augmentation necessary to bring these leads up to the size of leads I, II, and III.

Lead aVL (+) is at _____°.   −30

Lead aVF (+) is at _____°.   +90

Lead aVR (+) is at _____°.   −150

Leads aVR + aVL + aVF=0

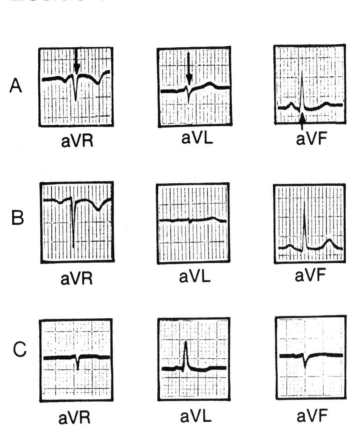

The summation of leads I, II, and III
is: _____

lead I + lead III = lead II

The summation of leads aVR, aVL and aVF
is: _____

leads aVR + aVL + aVF = 0

These relationships are of importance in the
evaluation of every electrocardiogram.

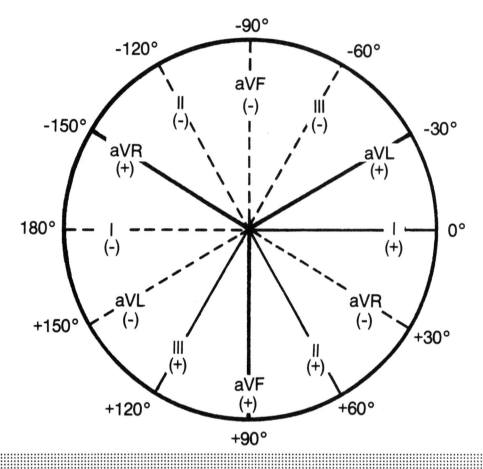

Formation of Hexaxial System
I, II, III, aVR, aVL, aVF

These six leads form a *hexaxial* system. The solid line represents the *positive* half of each lead; the broken line represents the *negative* half. The part of the circle used most frequently in clinical electrocardiography contains

LEAD	DEGREES
positive aVL	−30°
positive I	0°
negative aVR	+30°
positive II	+60°
positive aVF	+90°
positive III	+120°

Note that *negative* aVR at +30° is used. Positive aVR is a −150°.

Throughout the text, the degrees of the positive leads are labeled with or without the + sign (e.g., 60° or + 60°). Every negative lead is labeled with the − sign (e.g., −30°).

Practice

Place the appropriate leads and degrees on the following diagram.

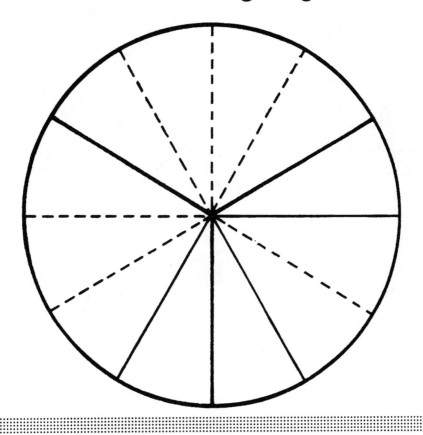

Answer:

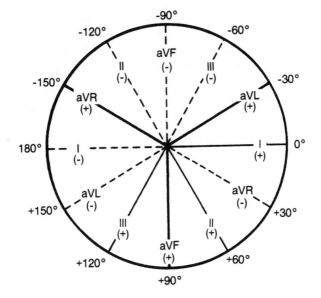

The Cardiac Vectors

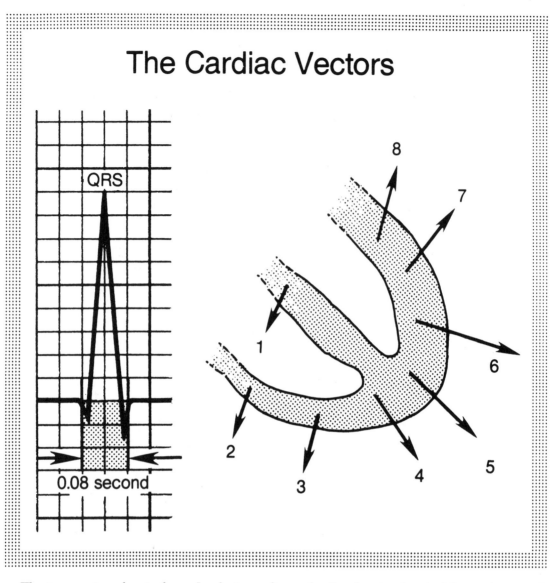

The term *vector* refers to force. In electrocardiography it refers to electrical force. A vector is represented by an arrow where both size and direction are easily demonstrated. Within a period of 0.08 sec. both ventricles are depolarized. During this single QRS interval, sequential instantaneous vectors are generated. The greater the muscle mass, the bigger the arrow will be.

The vectorial arrow represents both _____   size
and _____ .   direction

Both ventricles are normally depolarized within a period
of _____ sec.   0.08

Mean QRS Vector
Mean Electrical Axis of QRS
"Axis" of QRS

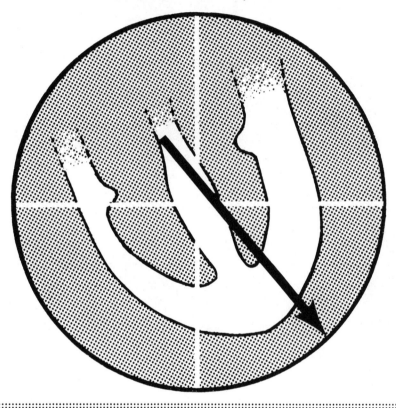

The *mean QRS vector* is the resultant, or the mean vector, of all the instantaneous vectors within a single QRS interval. We often refer to the mean QRS vector, mean T vector, and mean P vector in the study of electrocardiography. Because of common usage, the terms *mean electrical axis, electrical axis,* or simply *"axis"* of the QRS, T, and P are used.

The resultant of all the instantaneous vectors within a single QRS
interval is known as the _____ _____ _____ .   mean QRS vector

The mean vector of the QRS, T, and P wave is often called
the _____ of the QRS, T, and P, respectively.   "axis"

Determination of Mean QRS Vector

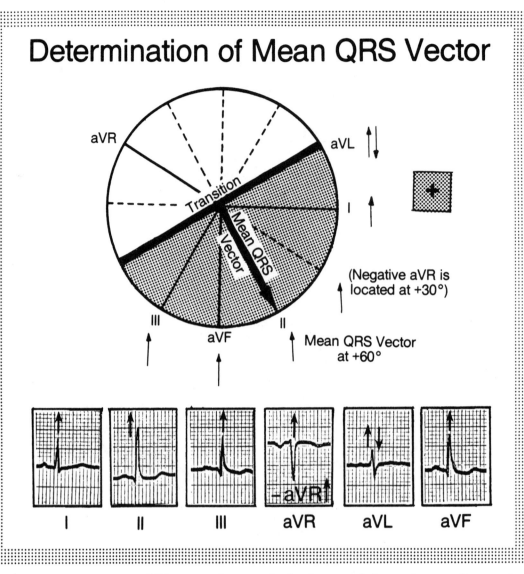

To determine the mean QRS vector, line up the leads around the circle according to their positivity or negativity. Note that *negative* aVR is at +30°; lead aVR must therefore be inverted before being placed on the circle. Lead aVL is neither predominantly positive nor predominantly negative; the transition is therefore through lead aVL. The *mean QRS vector* is at right angles to the transitional zone on the positive side. In this electrocardiogram the *transitional zone* is at −30° and the mean QRS vector is at 60° (large arrow). The shaded area in the circle is the positive half.

To determine the mean QRS vector on the electrocardiogram,
line up the leads around the circle according to
their _____ or _____ .   positivity negativity

The mean QRS vector is at right angles to
the _____ zone on   transitional
the _____ side.   positive

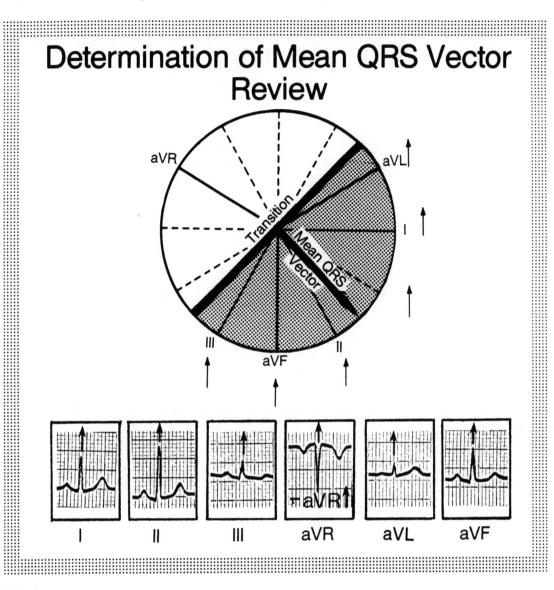

Review

To determine the mean QRS vector, the following steps should be taken sequentially.

1. Line up all six leads on the circle according to their positivity or negativity, from −30° to +120°. Lead aVR must be inverted at +30°.
2. Draw the transition, dividing the circle into positive and negative halves.
3. The mean QRS vector is at right angles to the transition on the positive side.

In this electrocardiogram the mean QRS vector is approximately 45° (large arrow). On the next three pages, practice this determination and then check answers below.

Practice
Locate Mean QRS Vector

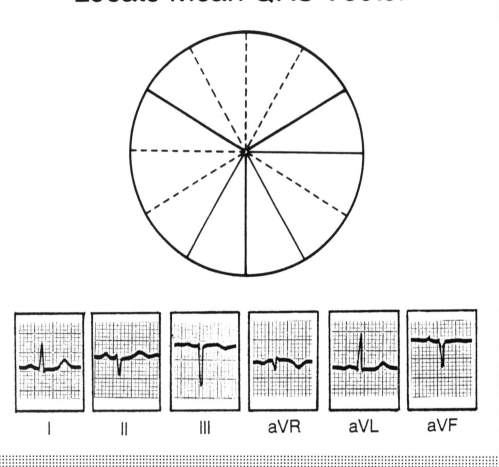

Answer:

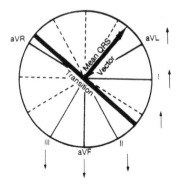

Practice
Locate Mean QRS Vector

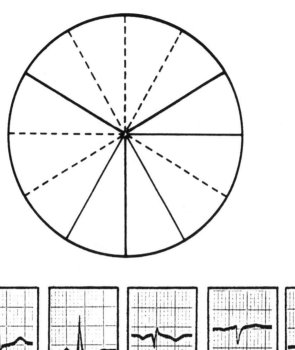

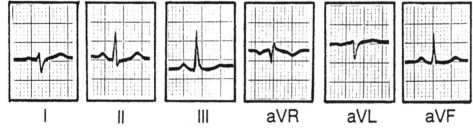

| I | II | III | aVR | aVL | aVF |

Answer:

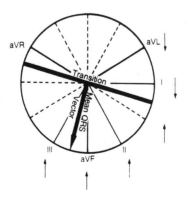

Practice
Locate Mean QRS Vector

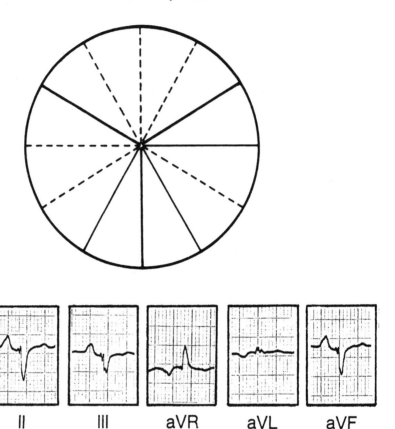

| I | II | III | aVR | aVL | aVF |

Answer:

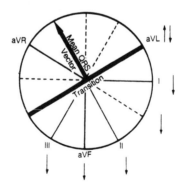

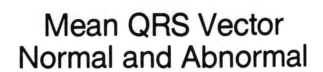

Mean QRS Vector
Normal and Abnormal

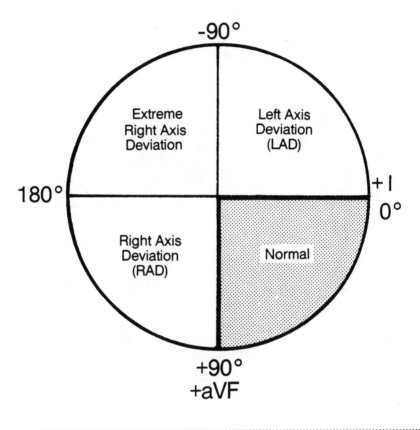

In the normal adult the mean QRS vector is usually between 0° and 90°, that is, the mean QRS vector is normally between leads I and aVF (shaded area). From 0° to −90° is *left axis deviation (LAD)* and from *90° to 180°* is *right axis deviation (RAD)*. The area from −90° to 180° has usually been described as *extreme right axis deviation*.

The normal adult mean QRS vector is from _____° to _____°.　　0 +90
LAD is from _____° to _____°.　　0 −90
RAD is from _____° to _____°.　　+90 180

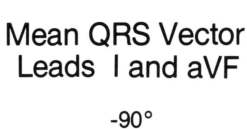

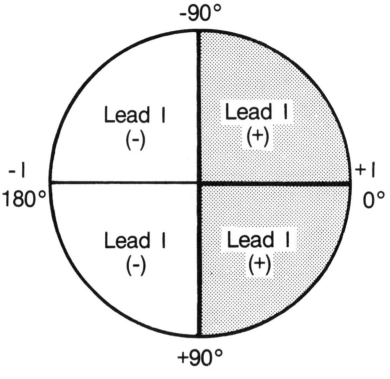

To quickly determine the quadrant in which the mean QRS vector is located, we need to examine leads I and aVF. Because these leads are at right angles to each other, the quadrant in which a mean QRS vector is located may be easily found by using these two leads. The entire left (shaded) half of the circle is *positive* for lead I. Therefore, if the QRS complex is *positive* in lead I, the mean QRS vector is either normal or deviated to the left. If the QRS complex is *negative* in lead I, we have right axis or extreme right axis deviation.

If the QRS complex in lead I:
is positive, the mean QRS vector is either _____ or   normal
deviated to the _____ .   left

is negative, the mean QRS vector is deviated either to   right
the _____ or the _____ _____ .   extreme right

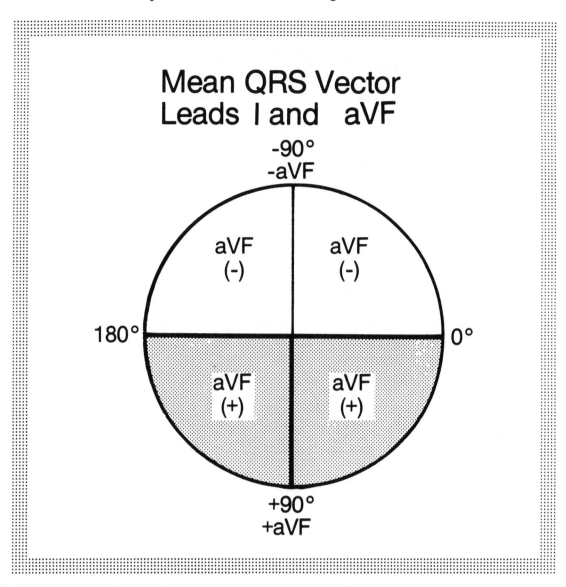

The entire lower half (shaded) of the circle is *positive* for lead aVF and the upper half is *negative* for lead aVF. Therefore, if the QRS complex is *positive* in lead aVF, the mean QRS vector is either normal or deviated to the right. If the QRS complex is *negative,* we have left axis deviation or extreme right axis deviation.

If the QRS complex in lead aVF:

is positive, the mean QRS vector is either _____ or deviated   normal
to the _____ .   right

is negative, we have either _____   LAD
or _____ _____ .   extreme RAD

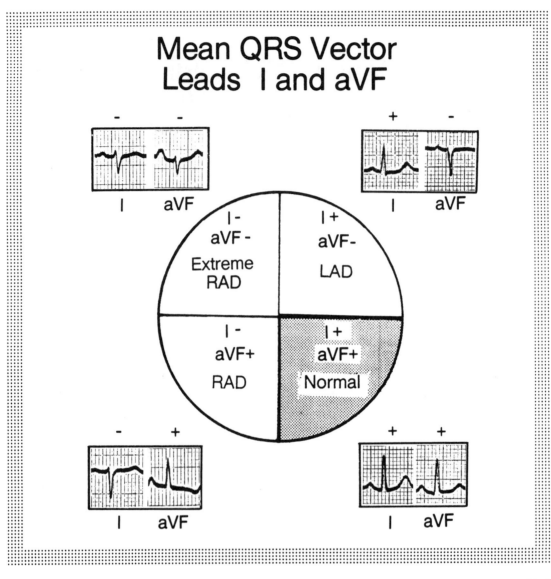

By utilizing both leads I and aVF, we can localize the quadrant containing the mean QRS vector. If both leads I and aVF are *positive,* the mean QRS vector is normal (shaded area). Describe leads I and aVF in *left axis deviation, right axis deviation,* and *extreme right axis deviation.*

Positivity or negativity of the QRS complexes in leads I and aVF in determination of the mean QRS vector

+I, −aVF = _____   LAD
−I, +aVF = _____   RAD
−I, −aVF = _____ _____   extreme RAD

Mean T Vector

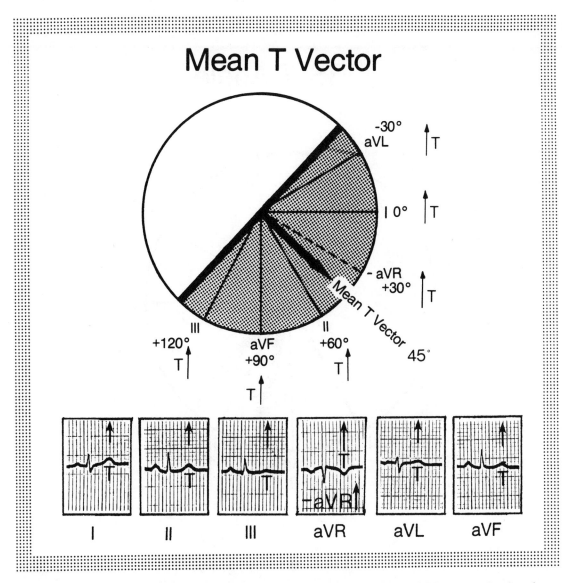

The *mean T vector* is determined in the same manner as the mean QRS vector. In the above illustration the T waves are positive in all the leads, including negative aVR (shaded area). The transition for the T wave bypasses all the leads. The mean T vector is perpendicular to the transition, on the positive side, at approximately 45° (large arrow).

The mean T vector is determined in the same manner as the mean _____ vector.

QRS

When all the T waves are positive (including −aVR), the mean T vector is at _____ .

45°

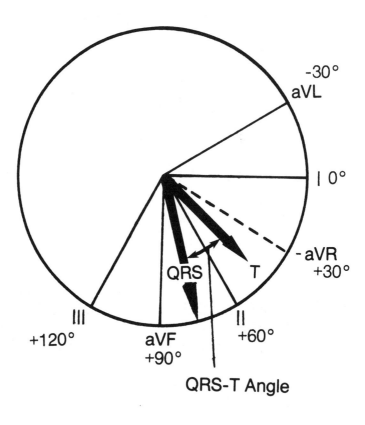

QRS-T Angle

The angle formed between the mean QRS vector and the mean T vector is a sensitive method for relating the forces of ventricular depolarization to the forces of ventricular repolarization. In the normal adult the *QRS-T angle* is rarely greater than 60° and often less than 45°. In the above illustration, using the same electrocardiogram as on the previous page, we find the QRS-T angle to be 30°.

The _____ angle relates the forces of ventricular depolarization to the forces of ventricular repolarization.   QRS-T

In the normal adult, the QRS-T angle is rarely greater than _____ .   60°

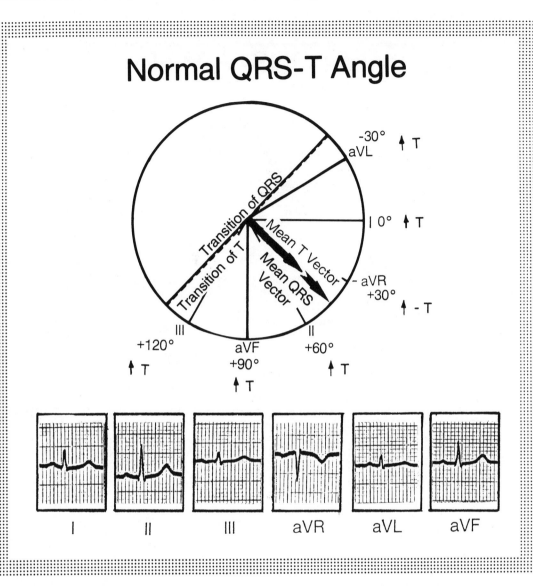

All the QRS complexes are positive, as are all the T waves. The mean QRS vector and the mean T vector are superimposed, thereby forming a very narrow, if any, angle between them. For the QRS-T angle to be normally narrow, the T wave should have the *same* orientation as the QRS complex (e.g., both positive) in leads I, II, and aVF. If not, stop and calculate. It may still be within normal limits. On the next two pages are examples of a wide and a very wide QRS-T angle.

If the QRS complexes and T waves have the same orientation in leads _____ , _____ , and _____ (e.g. positive), the QRS-T angle is normally narrow.   I II aVF

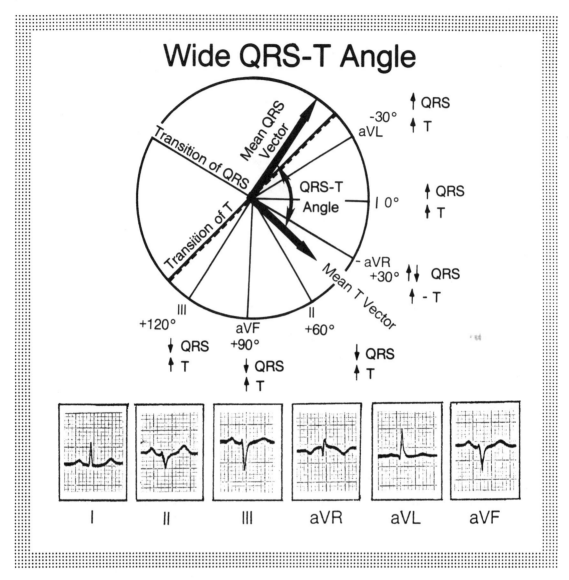

All the T waves are *positive* (including negative aVR), with the mean T vector at 45°. Owing to the marked left axis deviation of the mean QRS vector (−60°), a wide angle is formed between the mean QRS vector and the mean T vector (105°). Note: The T wave does not have the same orientation as the QRS complex in leads II and aVF.

The QRS complexes and T waves do not have the same orientation in leads II and aVF. The QRS-T angle is therefore abnormally _____.   wide

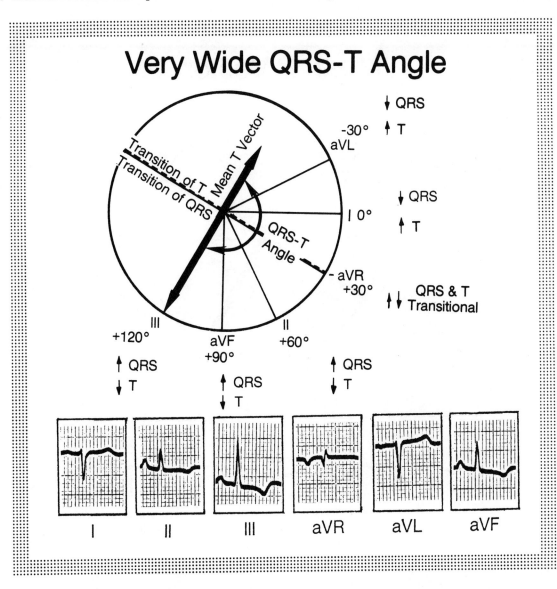

The transitional zone for both the mean QRS vector and the mean T vector is at lead aVR. In all other leads the QRS deflections are opposite the T wave deflections. The right axis deviation of the mean QRS vector (120°) and the left axis deviation (−60°) of the mean T vector result in a very wide QRS-T angle (180°).

Except for sharing the transition at lead aVR, the QRS complex and T waves are opposite in orientation in all other leads. The QRS-T angle is therefore abnormally wide at _____ .   180°

Mean P Vector

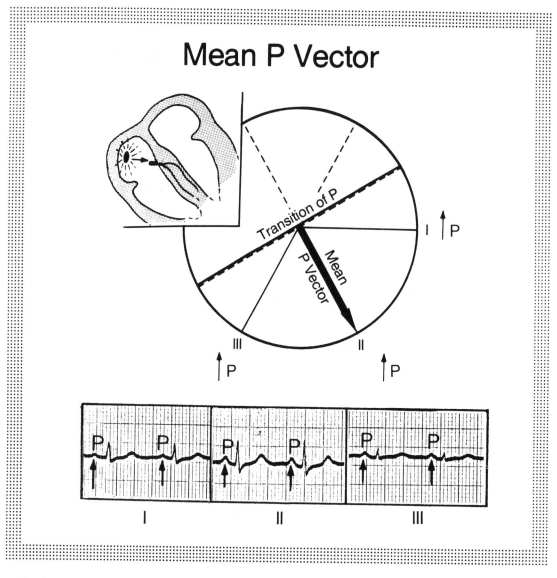

To find the *mean P vector,* use the same approach as for the mean QRS and T vectors. Note above that the mean P vector is along the axis of lead II at 60°. The normal range for the mean P vector is between 0° and +90°, usually between +15° and +75°. Therefore, the P waves in normal sinus rhythm are usually *positive* in leads I, II, and aVF.

In the normal:

The mean P vector is usually _____ to _____ .   **15° 75°**

the P waves are usually positive in leads _____ , _____ ,   **I II**
and _____ .

aVF

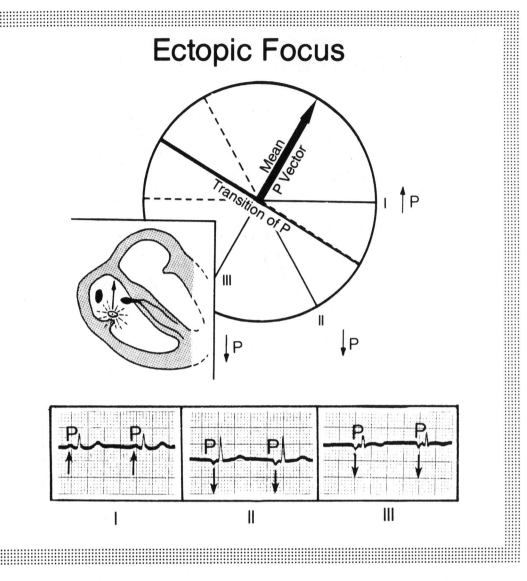

Ectopic Focus

The P wave is *positive* in lead I but *negative* in leads II and III. The transition is therefore between leads I and II, with an abnormal deviation of the mean P vector. Thus, the electrical impulse is not from the S-A node, but from some other focus; it is from an *ectopic focus* representing an abnormal sequence of atrial depolarization.

A P wave that is positive in lead I but negative in leads II and aVF reveals an _____ focus, with an abnormal sequence of atrial depolarization.   ectopic

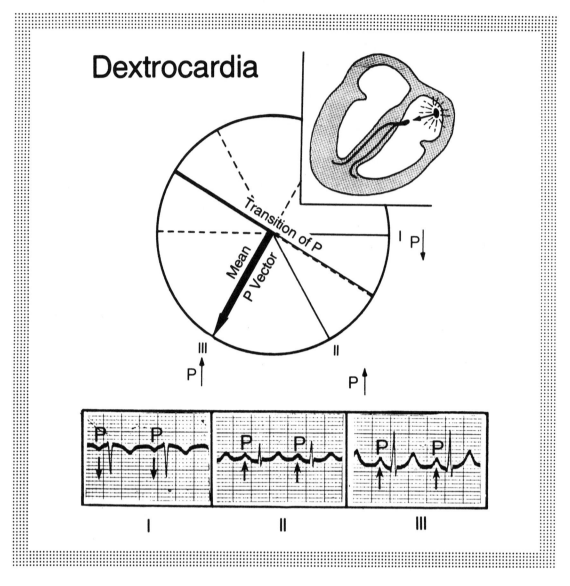

This electrocardiogram is from a patient with dextrocardia. The P wave is *negative* in lead I but *positive* in leads II and III. The mean P vector is deviated abnormally to the right. Another more common cause of a negative P wave in lead I is the reversal of electrodes in lead I (positive on the right arm and negative on the left).

The most common cause of a negative P wave in lead I is _____ arm leads.   reversed

A _____ P wave in lead _____ may indicate dextrocardia.   negative I

Heart Rate
Paper Speed = 25 mm./sec.

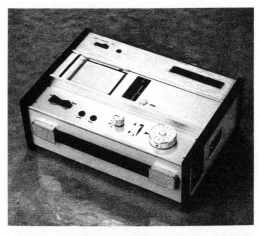

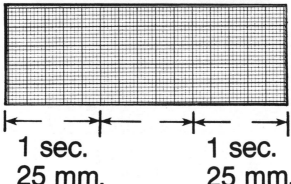

1 sec.   1 sec.
25 mm.   25 mm.

The determination of heart rate from the electrocardiogram depends on the speed of the paper when recording the electrocardiogram. The standard speed of the paper is *25 mm. (five large boxes) per sec.* Whenever the paper speed is changed, which is possible on most machines, it should be indicated on the electrocardiogram.

The standard electrocardiographic paper speed is _____ **mm. per sec.**   25

At the standard electrocardiographic paper speed, 5 large boxes
equal _____ _____ **.**   1 sec.

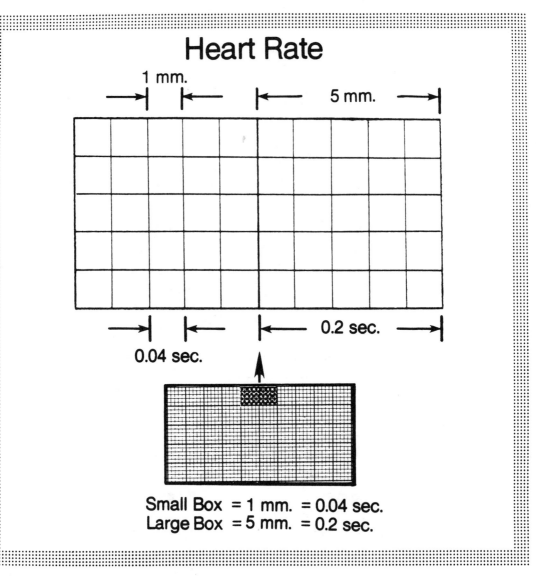

The electrocardiogram is recorded on lined paper that consists of large and small boxes. *Each large box measures 5 mm.* and *each small box 1 mm.* At the paper speed of 25 mm. per sec., *each large box represents 0.2 sec.* and *each small box 0.04 sec.*

Each large box on electrocardiographic paper measures _____ mm. and at standard paper speed, _____ sec.	5 0.2
Each small box on electrocardiographic paper measures _____ mm. and at standard paper speed, _____ sec.	1 0.04

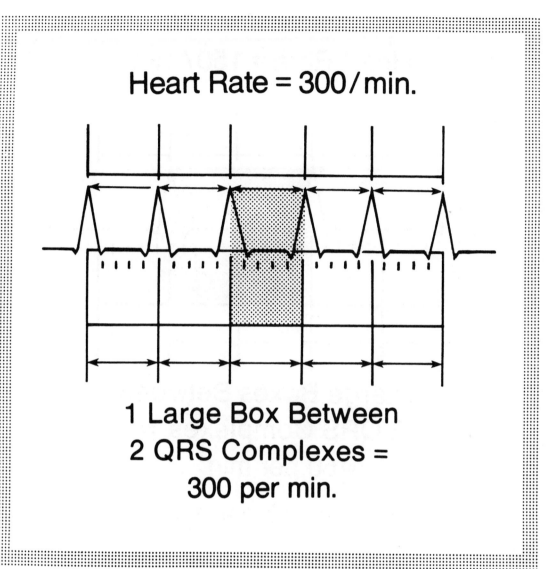

Heart Rate = 300 / min.

1 Large Box Between
2 QRS Complexes =
300 per min.

At the usual paper speed of 25 mm. per sec. (five large boxes), when the heart rate is *300 per min.,* the interval is *one large box (5 mm., 0.2 sec.) between two QRS complexes.* All that is necessary to determine heart rate when the rhythm is regular is to count the number of large boxes between two QRS complexes and divide into 300.

To determine heart rate when the rhythm is regular, _____ QRS   **two**
complexes are needed.

At standard electrocardiographic paper speed, one large box between two QRS
complexes equals a rate of _____ per min.   **300**

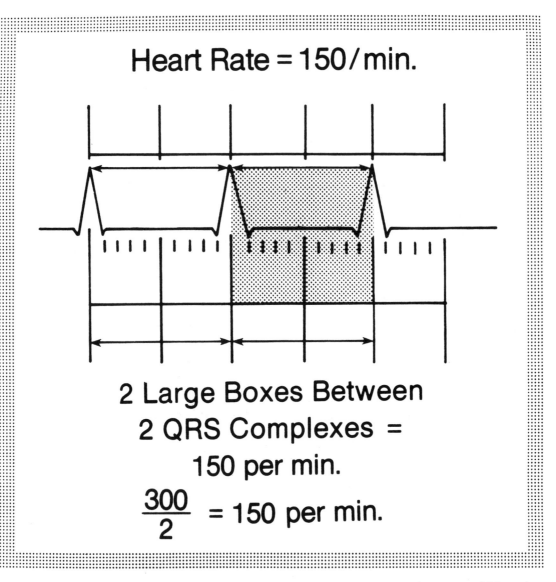

Heart Rate = 150/min.

2 Large Boxes Between
2 QRS Complexes =
150 per min.
$$\frac{300}{2} = 150 \text{ per min.}$$

When the heart rate is 150 per min., the interval is *two large boxes (0.4 sec.) between two QRS complexes (300/2)*. This determination is facilitated if you start the count with a QRS complex or P wave, whichever you are measuring, that falls on a heavy line.

Two large boxes on electrocardiographic paper measure _____ mm. and at standard paper speed, _____ sec.	10 0.4
At standard electrocardiographic paper speed, two large boxes between two QRS complexes equal a rate of _____ per min.	150

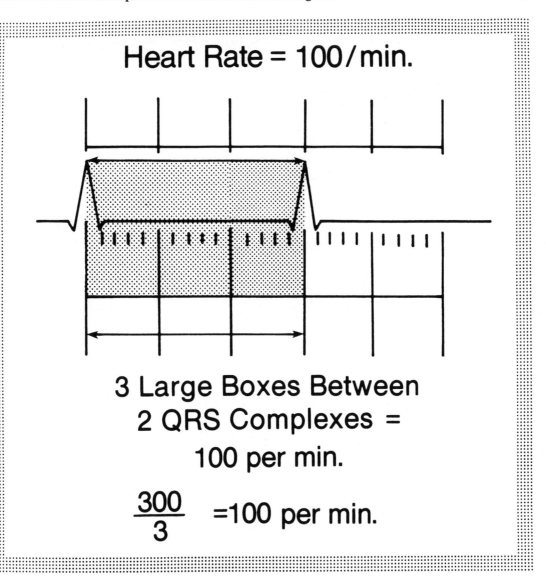

When the heart rate is 100 per min., the interval is *three large boxes (0.6 sec.) between two QRS complexes (300/3).*

Three large boxes on electrocardiographic paper measure _____ mm. and at standard paper speed, _____ sec.	15 0.6
At standard electrocardiographic paper speed, three large boxes between two QRS complexes equal a rate of _____ per min.	100

Practice
Determination of Heart Rate

Interval
(No. of Large Boxes)
Between
2 QRS Complexes   Rate/min.

1   =   _____

2   =   _____

3   =   _____

4   =   _____

5   =   _____

6   =   _____

7   =   _____

8   =   _____

9   =   _____

10   =   _____

Answers:

1	=	300 (300÷1)
2	=	150 (300÷2)
3	=	100 (300÷3)
4	=	75 (300÷4)
5	=	60 (300÷5)
6	=	50 (300÷6)
7	=	43 (300÷7)
8	=	38 (300÷8)
9	=	33 (300÷9)
10	=	30 (300÷10)

This relationship permits the determination of heart rate using only two QRS complexes when the rhythm is regular. Simply count the number of large boxes and any fraction, and divide into 300 for the heart rate. When the rhythm is irregular, you have to count numerous QRS complexes to arrive at the proper average, or use the method described on page 62.

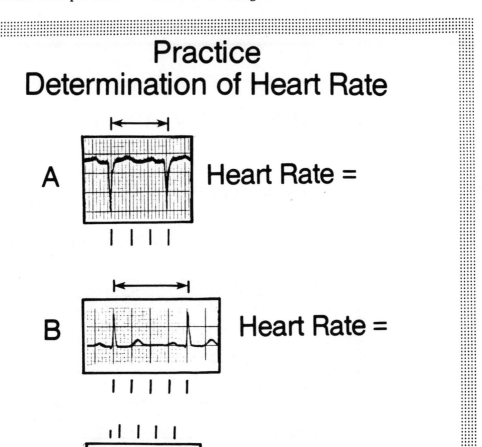

Practice
Determination of Heart Rate

A   Heart Rate =

B   Heart Rate =

C   Heart Rate =

Answers:

A. Three large boxes between two QRS complexes: heart rate = 100 per min. (300 ÷ 3 = 100).

B. Four large boxes between two QRS complexes: heart rate = 75 per min. (300 ÷ 4 = 75).

C. Three and a half large boxes between two QRS complexes: heart rate = 86 per min. (300 ÷ 3.5 = 86).

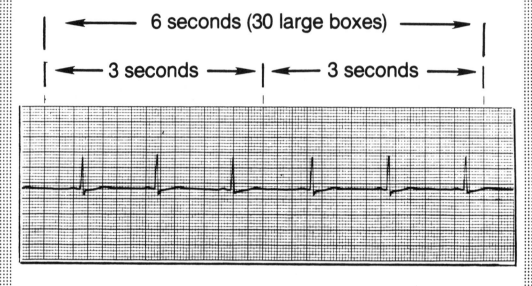

Heart Rate Determination
Another Method

← 6 seconds (30 large boxes) →

← 3 seconds → | ← 3 seconds →

QRS Complexes in 6 sec. x 10 = Heart Rate

Another method of determining heart rate is to utilize the 3-sec. markers (15 large boxes = 3 sec.) at the upper border of the electrocardiographic paper. Count the number of QRS complexes in a 6-sec. period and multiply by 10 for the rate per min. Within the 6-sec. period above are six QRS complexes. Therefore, the heart rate is 6 × 10 = 60 per min. This method is especially useful when the rhythm is not regular. Very often, the electrocardiographic paper has been cut down so that the marks are not evident. In that case, count 30 large boxes (6 sec.) and the number of QRS complexes within the 30 boxes and multiply by 10.

Electrocardiographic paper has _____-sec. markers; _____large   3   15 boxes equal 3 sec. at standard paper speed.

To determine heart rate, count the number of QRS complexes in a 6-sec. period and multiply by _____ .   **10**

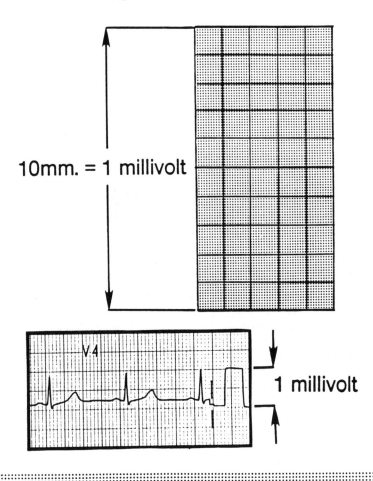

Electrocardiographic Standardization

10mm. = 1 millivolt

V.4

1 millivolt

The usual standardization on the electrocardiogram of 1 millivolt results in a deflection of two large boxes (10 mm.). The standardization is essential to properly evaluate the size of the deflections even if the electrocardiogram has been enlarged or reduced in size.

The usual electrocardiographic standardization of 1 millivolt results
in a deflection of _____ large boxes.   two

This standardization allows the comparison of electrocardiograms
even if the electrocardiogram has been _____   enlarged
or _____ _____ _____ .   reduced in size

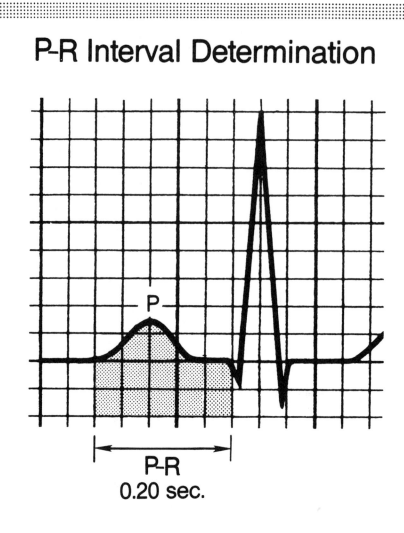

P-R Interval Determination

P

P-R
0.20 sec.

The P-R interval (from the beginning of the P wave to the beginning of the QRS complex) is 0.20 sec. (five small boxes or one large box). *The normal P-R interval is from 0.12 to 0.20 sec.* This is an important measurement, since an abnormal prolongation represents a delay in the transmission of the electrical impulse from the atria to the ventricles. A shorter than normal P-R interval (0.1 sec. or less) has been associated with various rhythm disturbances.

The normal P-R interval is _____ to _____ sec.

0.12 0.20

A prolonged P-R interval represents a _____ in the transmission of the impulse from the _____ to the _____ .

delay

atria ventricles

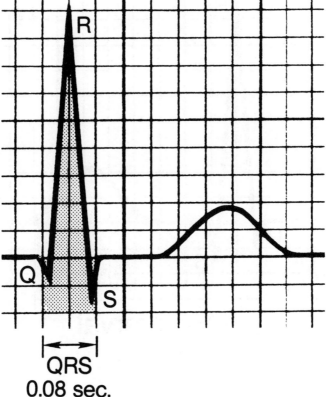

QRS Interval Determination

The QRS interval is 0.08 sec. (two small boxes). *The normal interval for ventricular depolarization is up to 0.1 sec.* Abnormal prolongation represents an intraventricular conduction disturbance. QRS interval prolongation is seen in right and left bundle branch block. These are studied in a later chapter.

The normal QRS interval is up to _____ sec.   0.1

An abnormal _____ of the QRS interval represents an   prolongation
intraventricular conduction disturbance.

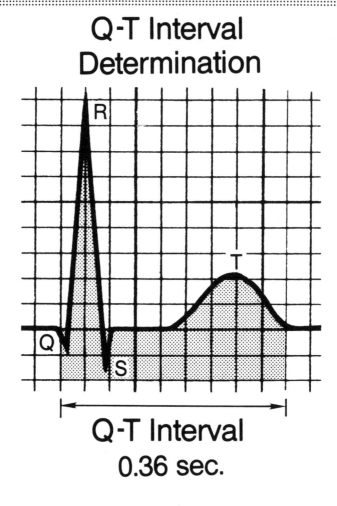

The ventricular repolarization process is longer at the lower rates, which is reflected in the longer Q-T interval at the lower rates.

Heart Rate (beats per min.)	Q-T Interval (sec.)
40	0.46
60	0.39
80	0.35
100	0.31
120	0.29
140	0.26
160	0.25

The Q-T interval:

is rate _____.   dependent

is decreased at the _____ rates.   higher

Normal Sinus Rhythm

1. Normal Mean P Vector (to the left and inferior - upright P waves in leads I and aVF or I and II.

2. Each P wave must be followed by a QRS complex and each QRS complex must be preceded by a P wave.

3. The normal P-R interval (from the beginning of the P wave to the beginning of the QRS complex) is rarely greater than 0.2 sec. (one large box) in duration. The normal range is 0.12 to 0.2 sec. and is constant from beat to beat.

4. The rate is constant between 60 and 100 beats per minute.

In order to describe the rhythm of the heart as *sinus rhythm* (the impulse originating in the sinoatrial node, which is the normal pacemaker of the heart) without qualifications, the above requirements must be met.

In normal sinus rhythm:

each _____ _____ must be followed by a _____ _____ and   P wave

each _____ _____ must be preceded by a _____ _____.   QRS complex

QRS complex

P wave

the rate is constant between _____ and _____ per minute.   60 100

> The ladder diagram or "laddergram" is a useful aid in the study of normal and abnormal rhythms of the heart. It is explained and illustrated on pages 356 and 357.

The Frontal Plane

Superior

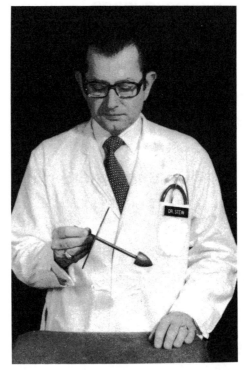

Right   Left

Inferior

The six electrocardiographic leads studied heretofore—I, II, III, aVR, aVL, and aVF—are leads in the *frontal plane*. The boundaries of the frontal plane are *superior, inferior, right, and left.*

We are still missing the third dimension, since the cardiac vector is three-dimensional.

Leads I, II, III, aVR, aVL, and aVF comprise the _____plane.	frontal
The boundaries of the frontal plane are _____, _____, _____, and _____ .	superior inferior right left

Frontal Plane Vectors

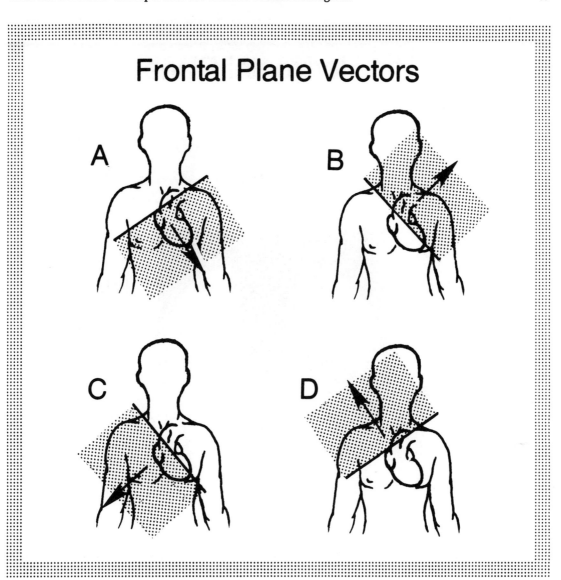

When the mean QRS, T, and P vectors were indicated by an arrow, only *two* dimensions in space could be described.

A. The arrow points to the _____ _____ _____ .   left and inferiorly
B. The arrow points to the _____ _____ _____ .   left and superiorly
C. The arrow points to the _____ _____ _____ .   right and inferiorly
D. The arrow points to the _____ _____ _____ .   right and superiorly

The Horizontal Plane

Posterior

Right 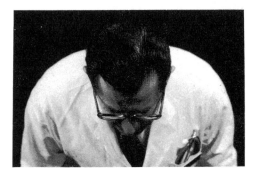 Left

Anterior

In order to provide the third dimension in space to describe the cardiac vectors, the *horizontal* plane must be added. The boundaries of the horizontal plane are *anterior, posterior, right,* and *left.* After many years and many trials, the chest or precordial leads were established (page 71). Still later, measurements of the cardiac vectors in the horizontal plane were shown to be possible.

The _____ plane was added to provide the third   horizontal
dimension in space to describe the cardiac vectors.

The boundaries of the horizontal plane
are _____ , _____ ,   anterior posterior
_____ , and _____ .   right left

Precordial Leads V₁-V₆

A

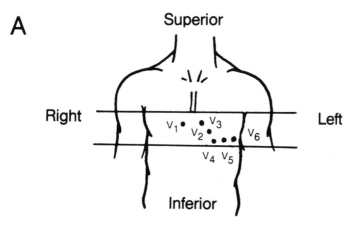

B

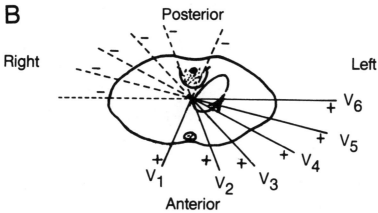

A. Precordial electrode positions are as follows:
  V_1: Fourth intercostal space to the right of the sternum
  V_2: Fourth intercostal space to the left of the sternum
  V_3: Midway between V_2 and V_4
  V_4: Fifth intercostal space—midclavicular line
  V_5: Anterior axillary line—horizontal level of V_4
  V_6: Midaxillary line—horizontal level of V_4
B. QRS loop in the horizontal plane.

Leads V_1 to V_6 comprise the _____ __ _____ leads.   precordial or chest

Mean QRS Vector in Three Dimensions

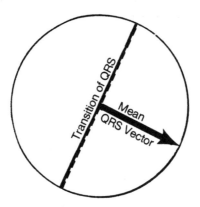

Mean QRS Vector—Left and Inferior

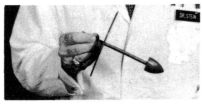 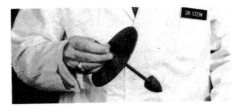

A   B

A.   In two dimensions, the disk is seen as a line with an arrow.
B.   In three dimensions, the full disk is seen with the posterior tilt of the arrow.

While studying the mean QRS vector in the frontal plane, we were accustomed to seeing a line and an arrow. We had not really been looking at a transitional *line* but at a *disk* dividing the body into positive and negative areas. The circumference of this disk, viewed on end, appeared to be a line (A). In a three-dimensional view, as seen in B, the disk and arrow are tilted slightly posteriorly to show that we are not actually looking at a line, but at a disk.

In studying the mean QRS vector in the frontal plane, the arrow represents the mean QRS vector, and perpendicular to it is a _____, representing the transition.

line

In the three-dimensional study we see that the transitional line is really a _____, dividing the body into positive and negative zones.

disk

Vectorial Concept in Three Dimensions

Vector Model

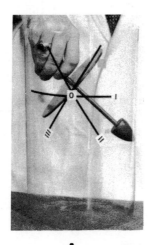

A

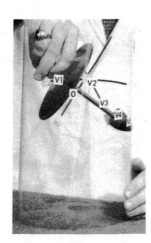

B

A. Frontal leads   B. Horizontal leads

The vector model may be used to better visualize the cardiac vector in three dimensions. The lines in A, representing the *frontal* plane, are leads I, II, and III. The precordial leads in B, representing the *horizontal* plane, are leads V_1 to V_6. The zero on the frontal plane and the zero on the horizontal plane line up, and they line up with the center point of the disk. *We can rotate the disk only through the zero point,* which limits its motion. This method facilitates the understanding of the general vectorial concept in three dimensions.

To better visualize the cardiac vector in three dimensions,
a _____ _____ may be used.   vector model

The vector model consists of the _____ plane leads on one side   frontal
and the _____ plane leads on the other.   horizontal

Stepwise Determination of Mean QRS Vector in Three Dimensions

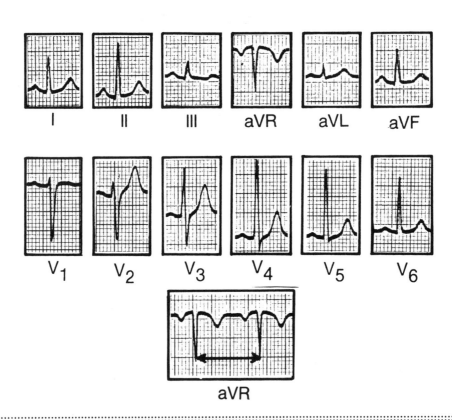

This electrocardiogram is analyzed on the next three pages as to the mean QRS vector in three dimensions. We will first determine the mean QRS vector in the frontal plane, using leads I, II, III, aVR, aVL, and aVF. Then we will examine the contribution of the precordial (chest) leads, V_1 to V_6, to our understanding of the mean QRS vector in three dimensions.

**Determine the mean QRS vector in the frontal plane on the next page
and check your answer at the bottom of the page.**

The heart rate is _____ per min.   88 (300/3.4)

Mean QRS Vector
Frontal Plane
Practice

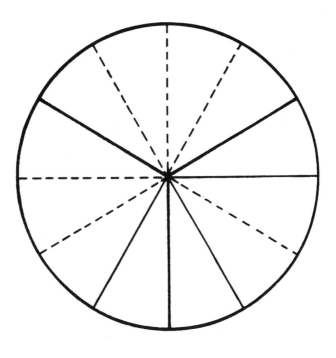

Answer:

All six leads are positive, remembering to invert lead aVR. The transitional zone bypasses all of the leads, and the mean QRS vector falls between leads II and aVR, to the *left* and *inferiorly* in the frontal plane. The disk and arrow, held to the left and inferiorly, do not actually appear as a disk and an arrow but rather as a line and an arrow.

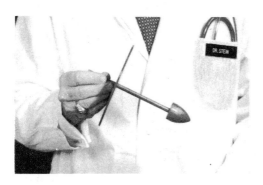

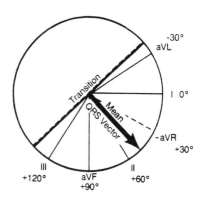

Vector Model
Frontal and Horizontal Leads

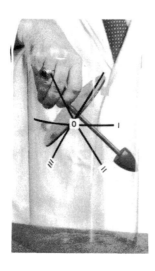

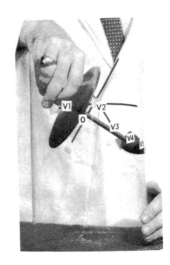

A

B

A. Frontal Plane
Leads I, II, III

B. Horizontal Plane
Leads V_1-V_6

Using our vector model in A we see leads I, II, and III, and the vector is to the *left* and *inferior*. In B, on the other side of the model, we have a representation of the horizontal plane. *If there were no anterior-posterior rotation,* if the vector were simply to the *left* and *inferior,* lead V_1 would be *negative.* V_1 is the only precordial lead on the negative side of the disk. The arrow side of the disk is the positive side.

As depicted in B, leads V_2, V_3, V_4, V_5, and V_6 would all be positive. Is this the case in the electrocardiogram on page 74?

No, lead V_2 is also predominantly negative.

Mean QRS Vector in Three Dimensions

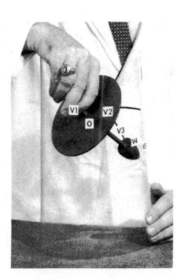

Left, Inferior, and Posterior

On looking again at page 74, we see that not only lead V_1 but also V_2 is *negative*. Leads V_3, V_4, V_5, and V_6 are *positive*. The transition in the horizontal plane is between leads V_2 and V_3. How do we make our model reflect the electrocardiographic inscription? We must tilt the disk so that the arrow faces *posteriorly*. In this position both leads V_1 and V_2 are negative. Leads V_3 through V_6 are positive.

The mean QRS vector, in three dimensions, is to the *left, inferior,* and *posterior.* This describes the normal adult mean QRS vector.

**The normal mean QRS vector in the adult is to the _____ , _____ ,   left inferior
and _____.**   posterior

> Older terms, less commonly used today, described the electrical position of the heart. These included the terms horizontal, vertical, semihorizontal, semivertical, and intermediate. It is much more common to state that the mean electrical axes are 0°, 45°, or 90° than to refer to those hearts as horizontal, intermediate, or vertical, respectively. Please refer to pages 358 and 359 for the illustration of the terms clockwise and counterclockwise rotation.

Stepwise Determination of Mean QRS Vector in Three Dimensions

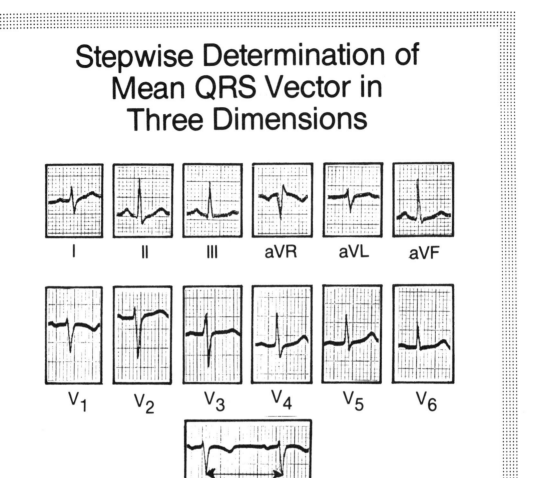

As we did with the previous electrocardiogram, we will analyze the mean QRS vector in three dimensions on the next three pages.

To summarize, whether the mean QRS vector is *left and inferior, left and superior, right and inferior,* or *right and superior* is determined by the *frontal plane leads,* I, II, III, aVR, aVL, and aVF. Whether the mean QRS vector is *anterior* or *posterior* must be determined from the *horizontal plane leads,* V_1 to V_6.

Determine the mean QRS vector in the frontal plane and check your answer on the next page.

The heart rate is _____ **per min.**   71 (300/4.2)

Mean QRS Vector
Frontal Plane
Practice

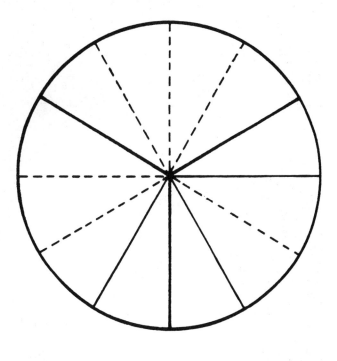

Answer:

In the frontal plane leads, I, II, III, aVR, aVL, and aVF, the transition is at lead I and the mean QRS vector is at 90°. The mean QRS vector in the frontal plane is neither to the left nor to the right. The arrow is pointing inferiorly.

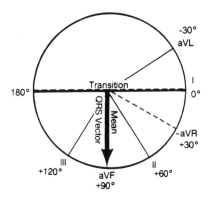

Mean QRS Vector at 90⁰
Using Vector Model

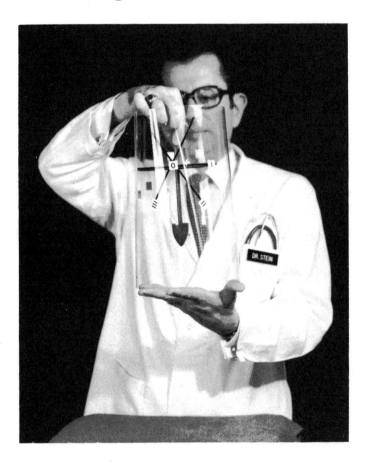

The vector model is very useful in enabling us to visualize the mean QRS vector in three dimensions. Here we are looking at the frontal plane leads, I, II, and III. The transition is at lead I, 0°, and the mean QRS vector is perpendicular to it at lead aVF, 90°.

Vector Model-Horizontal Plane

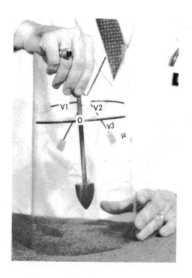

A

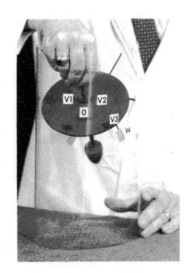

B

Horizontal Plane Leads V₁-V₆

A. If the mean QRS vector were directly inferior, neither anterior nor posterior, then leads V_1 and V_2 would both be negative and leads V_3 to V_6 would be positive.

B. The electrocardiogram on page 78, however, shows the transition to be between leads V_3 and V_4. In order to make lead V_3 negative on the vector model, we must tilt the arrow posteriorly. The mean QRS vector is, therefore, inferior and posterior in three dimensions.

In three dimensions, the mean QRS vector is _____
and _____ in this electrocardiogram.

inferior
posterior

Normal Mean QRS Vector in Three Dimensions

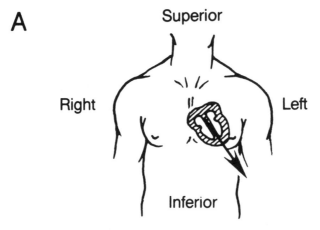

A

Superior

Right   Left

Inferior

Left, Inferior, and Posterior

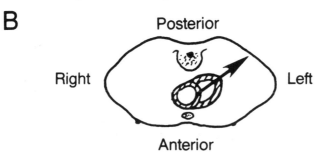

B

Posterior

Right   Left

Anterior

To summarize, the *normal* mean QRS vector in the *frontal* plane (A) is oriented to the *left* and *inferiorly.* In the *horizontal* plane (B), we see that it is also *posterior.*

The vector approach affords us a unifying concept in our understanding of the electrocardiogram. By visualizing the distribution of electrical potential in a three-dimensional way, a single picture actually indicates what we will find on the 12-lead electrocardiogram.

To review, before proceeding to the abnormal electrocardiogram on the next page, in the *normal adult,*the mean QRS vector is to the _____ , _____ , and _____ .

left inferior
posterior

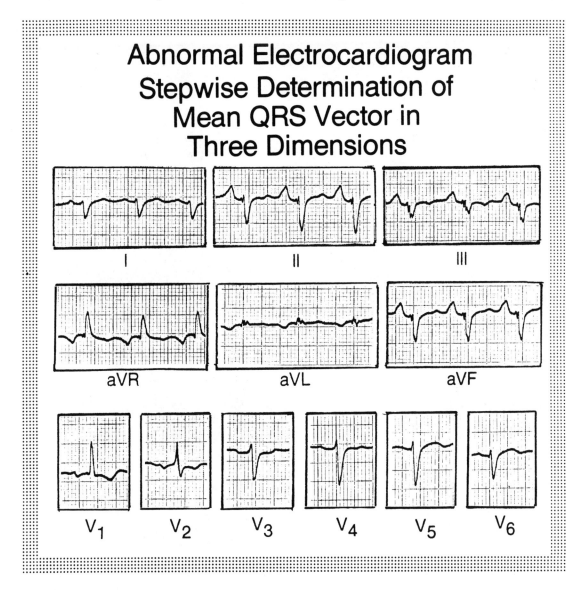

Abnormal Electrocardiogram
Stepwise Determination of Mean QRS Vector in Three Dimensions

This electrocardiogram is from a patient with chronic lung disease and resulting heart failure (cor pulmonale), with hypertrophy of the right atrium and right ventricle. These entities are studied in the next chapter. For the present, we will evaluate the mean QRS vector, as we have done in previous electrocardiograms.

Determine the mean QRS vector in the frontal plane and check your answer on the next page.

The heart rate is _____ per min.   100 (300/3)

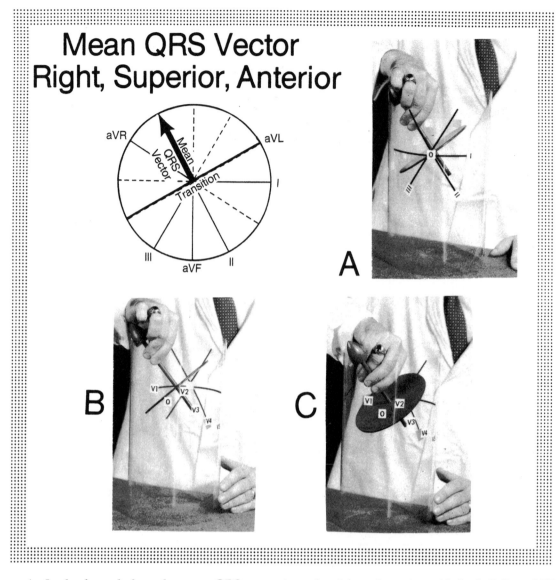

A. In the frontal plane the mean QRS vector is to the *right* and *superior,* with leads I, II, and III negative, facing away from the arrow side of the disk.

B. If the mean QRS vector were merely to the right and superior, lead V_1 would be positive and V_2 to V_6 would fall on the negative side of the disk.

C. The electrocardiogram (page 83), however, reveals that the transition is between leads V_2 and V_3. We must tilt the disk so the arrow points *anteriorly.*

In this patient, with chronic lung disease, the mean QRS vector is to the _____ , _____ , and _____ .   **right superior anterior**

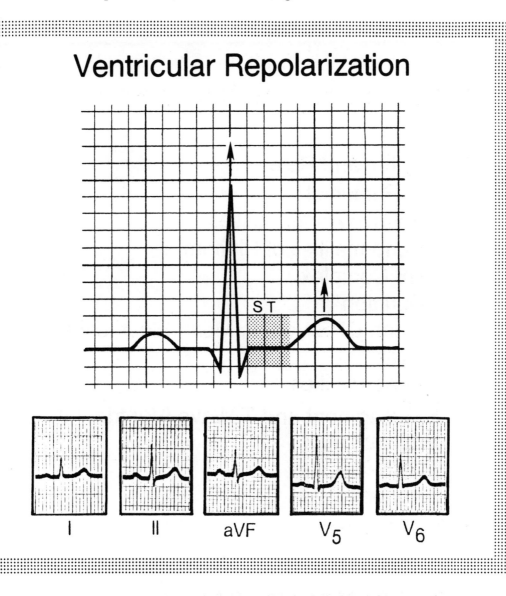

Before starting the complete analysis of the normal 12-lead electrocardiogram, the importance of the phase of ventricular repolarization must again be emphasized.

    1. The S-T segment is normally isoelectric, neither elevated nor depressed, at the same level as the resting baseline. The S-T segment may, however, slope upward toward a tall T wave.

    2. In order to have a normal QRS-T angle in *three dimensions,* the T wave is in the same direction (upward, positive, arrows above) as the QRS complex in leads I, II, aVF, V_5 and V_6.

The normal S-T segment is usually neither _____   elevated
nor _____ **.**   depressed

In the normal, three-dimensional QRS-T angle, the T wave is
usually in the same direction as the QRS complex in leads _____ **,**   I
_____ **,** _____ **,** _____ **, and** _____ **.**   II aVF V_5 V_6

Electrocardiographic Interpretation

1. Rhythm and Rate
   P-R Interval
   P Wave Abnormalities
   Abnormalities of Rhythm
2. QRS Complex
   Duration
   Mean QRS Vector, Mean Electrical Axis or "Axis"
   Abnormalities
3. S-T Segment and T Wave (Ventricular Repolarization)
   QRS-T Angle
   Abnormalities
4. Q-T Interval

Impression and Comment

Using all the information studied so far, we can analyze electrocardiograms according to the four steps enumerated above.

Practice
ECG Analysis

Practice
ECG Analysis

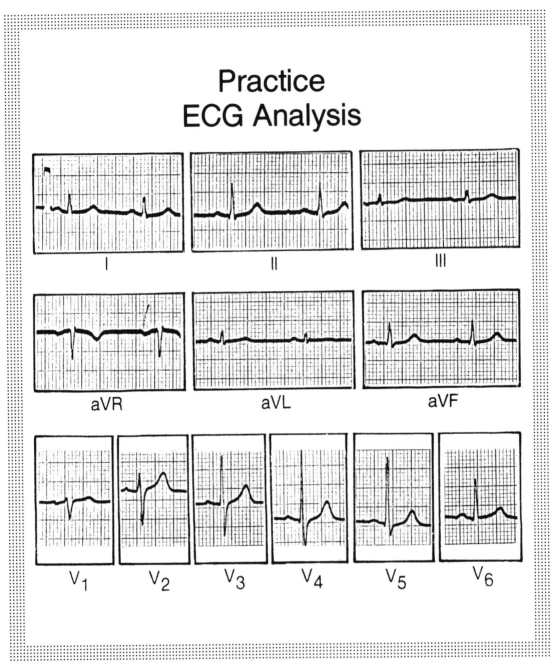

Using the four steps outlined on page 86, analyze this and the next electrocardiogram. After you have completed each analysis, compare with the review on the following page.

The patient is a healthy adult.

Analysis:

ECG ANALYSIS

1. Rhythm and rate
   Rhythm: sinus
   Rate: 65/min.
   P-R interval: 0.16 sec.
2. QRS complex
   Duration: 0.08 sec.
   Axis: + 45°
3. Ventricular repolarization
   S-T segment: neither significantly elevated nor depressed.
   T wave: QRS-T angle normal
4. Q-T interval: 0.38 sec.

Impression and Comment

Normal electrocardiogram

Practice
ECG Analysis

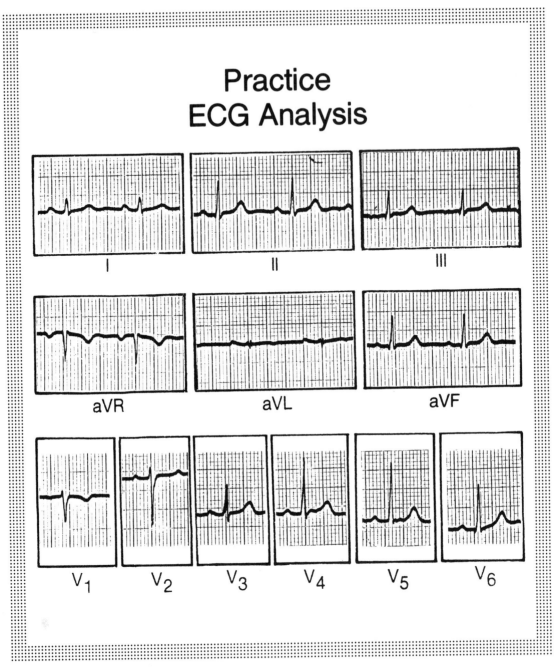

The patient is a healthy adult.

Analysis:

ECG ANALYSIS

1. Rhythm and rate
   Rhythm: sinus
   Rate: 75/min.
   P-R interval: 0.18 sec.
2. QRS complex
   Duration: 0.08 sec.
   Axis: + 60°
3. Ventricular repolarization
   S-T segment: neither significantly elevated nor depressed
   T wave: QRS-T angle normal
4. Q-T interval: 0.36 sec.

Impression and Comment

Normal electrocardiogram

Chapter 2

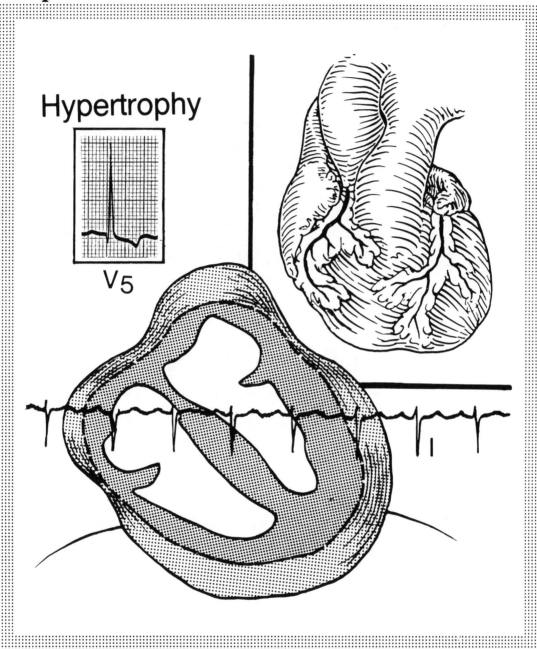

Hypertrophy

V5

Myocardial hypertrophy refers to an increase in the muscular wall thickness of a chamber of the heart. Hypertrophy is the result of *pressure overload,* where the heart pumps against increased resistance. This is seen in patients with aortic stenosis and systemic hypertension. The broader term, *enlargement,* also includes dilatation of a heart chamber, which is seen in *volume overload,* as in patients with aortic insufficiency and atrial septal defect. The appropriate chamber becomes dilated with the increased volume of blood. Hypertrophy and dilatation are often found together and may not be easily differentiated on the electrocardiogram.

Right Ventricular Hypertrophy

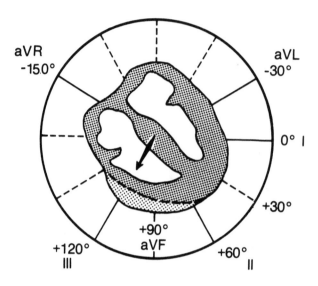

1. QRS Neg. in Lead I

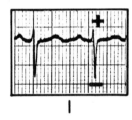

I

As the mean QRS vector (mean electrical axis of the QRS) shifts rightward, it faces *away* from lead I, inscribing a QRS complex in lead I that is *predominantly negative.* A predominantly negative QRS complex in lead I signifies right axis deviation. *Right axis deviation is a major electrocardiographic criterion of right ventricular hypertrophy.*

_____ _____ _____ is a major   **Right axis deviation**
electrocardiographic criterion of right ventricular hypertrophy.

Right axis deviation produces a
predominantly _____ **QRS complex in lead I.**   negative

Right Ventricular Hypertrophy

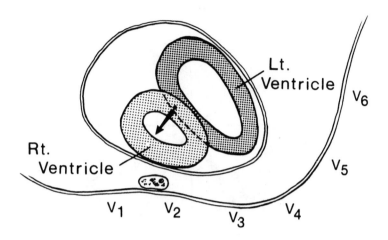

Lt. Ventricle

Rt. Ventricle

V_6

V_5

V_1 V_2 V_3 V_4

2. QRS Pos. in Lead V_1

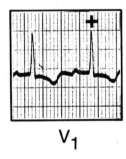

V_1

In right ventricular hypertrophy the mean QRS vector often shifts not only to the right, but also *anteriorly*. It therefore faces lead V_1, inscribing a predominantly *positive QRS complex in lead V_1*. *A predominantly positive QRS complex in lead V_1 is another major electrocardiographic criterion of right ventricular hypertrophy.*

In right ventricular hypertrophy the mean QRS vector often shifts to the right and _____.   anteriorly

This anterior mean QRS vector inscribes a predominantly _____QRS complex in lead V_1.   positive

Right Ventricular Hypertrophy

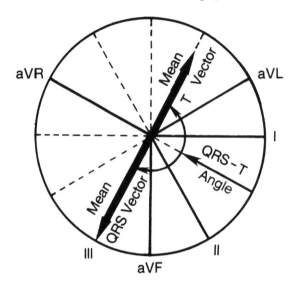

3. ST-T Abnormalities

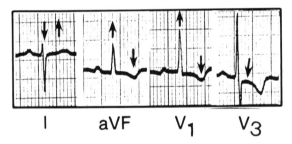

| I | aVF | V₁ | V₃ |

Ventricular repolarization (ST-T) abnormalities are frequently seen secondary to right ventricular hypertrophy. In the above electrocardiogram the QRS complexes and T waves are opposite in orientation. Where the QRS complex is positive the T wave is negative, and where the QRS is negative the T wave is positive. *The QRS-T angle is, therefore, very wide—180°.* S-T segment depression is seen in lead V_3.

S-T segment abnormalities and a _____ __ _____ QRS-T   wide or abnormal angle are commonly seen in right ventricular hypertrophy.

Right Ventricular Hypertrophy
Principal Criteria
Review

1. Neg. QRS in Lead I

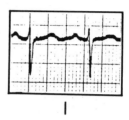

I

2. Pos. QRS in Lead V₁

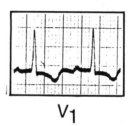

V₁

3. ST-T Abnormalities

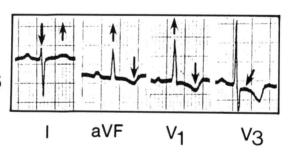

I   aVF   V₁   V₃

Review

In right ventricular hypertrophy the mean QRS vector often shifts *rightward* and *anteriorly,* inscribing both the *negative* QRS complex in lead I and the *positive* QRS complex in lead V₁. Ventricular repolarization (ST-T) abnormalities commonly accompany right ventricular hypertrophy. Causes of right ventricular hypertrophy include pulmonary disease and congenital heart disease.

To review, a mean QRS vector, oriented to the right and anteriorly inscribes a _____ QRS complex in lead I and a _____ QRS complex in lead V₁.

negative
positive

Causes of right ventricular hypertrophy include _____ _____ and _____ _____ _____.

pulmonary disease
congenital heart disease

> Additional criteria for right ventricular hypertrophy, including sensitivity and specificity, ventricular activation time and the intrinsicoid deflection, are found on pages 360 to 362.

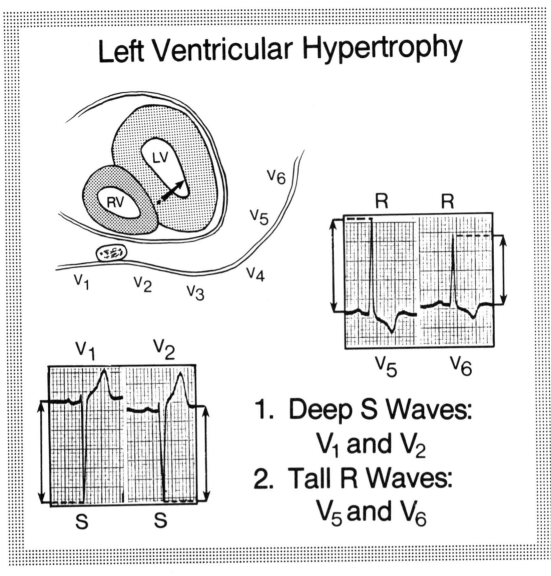

Left Ventricular Hypertrophy

1. Deep S Waves: V_1 and V_2
2. Tall R Waves: V_5 and V_6

In left ventricular hypertrophy the mean QRS vector, which is normally oriented to the left, inferiorly, and posteriorly, is markedly accentuated, inscribing *deep S waves* in the right precordial leads (V_1 and V_2) and *tall R waves* in the left precordial leads (V_5 and V_6).

In left ventricular hypertrophy:

the normal mean QRS vector, which is oriented to	left
the _____, _____, and _____, is accentuated.	inferiorly posteriorly
deep _____ waves may be seen in the right precordial	S
leads and tall _____ waves in the left precordial leads.	R

Left Ventricular Hypertrophy

1. Magnitude Criteria

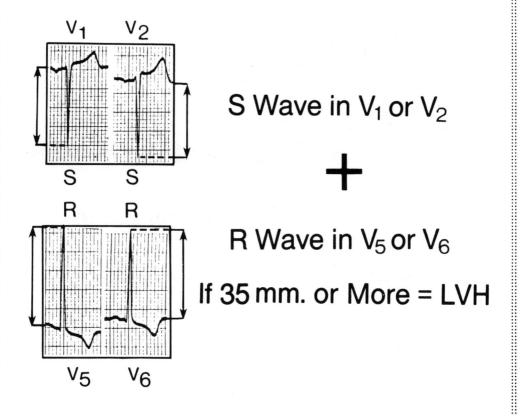

S Wave in V_1 or V_2

+

R Wave in V_5 or V_6

If 35 mm. or More = LVH

Increased magnitude of the QRS complex is the major electrocardiographic criterion of left ventricular hypertrophy in the adult. Because of the posterior orientation of the mean QRS vector in left ventricular hypertrophy, the increased magnitude is seen best in the precordial leads, V_1 to V_6. The diagnosis of left ventricular hypertrophy should not be made without evidence of increased magnitude. In addition, if any of the above leads (V_1, V_2, V_5, V_6) is 25 mm or more, alone (not in combination), left ventricular hypertrophy should be considered.

In left ventricular hypertrophy:

S_{V_1} or V_2 + R_{R_5} or V_6 ≥ _____ mm.   35

S_{V_1} or V_2 or R_{V_5} or V_6 ≥ _____ mm.   25

Left Ventricular Hypertrophy

2. ST-T Abnormalities

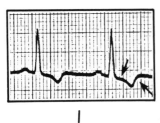

I

S-T Segment Depression and T Wave Inversion

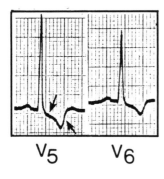

V₅   V₆

Ventricular repolarization (ST-T) abnormalities are frequently seen secondary to left ventricular hypertrophy. The *QRS-T angle is wide,* with the T waves inverted. Note the asymmetry of the inverted T waves. There is a slow downstroke, followed by a rapid upstroke. *S-T segment depression* is common.

In left ventricular hypertrophy:
the QRS-T angle is often _____ and the S-T   wide or abnormal
segment is _____ .   depressed

**The inverted T wave is
characteristically** _____ .   asymmetrical

Left Ventricular Hypertrophy
Principal Criteria
Review

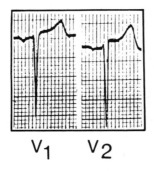

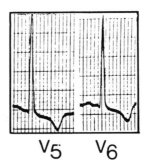

V₁   V₂   V₅   V₆

1. S_{V_1} or S_{V_2} + R_{V_5} or R_{V_6}

$> 35\,mm$

2. ST-T Abnormalities

Review

As the left ventricle hypertrophies, the mean QRS vector rotates more leftward and posteriorly. Left axis deviation may be seen in association with left ventricular hypertrophy, although it is not a major electrocardiographic criterion. Ventricular repolarization (ST-T) abnormalities are very common in left ventricular hypertrophy.

Note: The QRS magnitude criteria apply to *adults* of normal height and weight, because increased magnitude of the QRS complex without ST-T abnormalities may be seen in a *normal* youth.

_____ axis deviation may be seen in association with left ventricular hypertrophy.

Left

The magnitude criteria given for left ventricular hypertrophy apply to _____ .

adults

> See pages 363 to 365 for additional criteria for left ventricular hypertrophy.

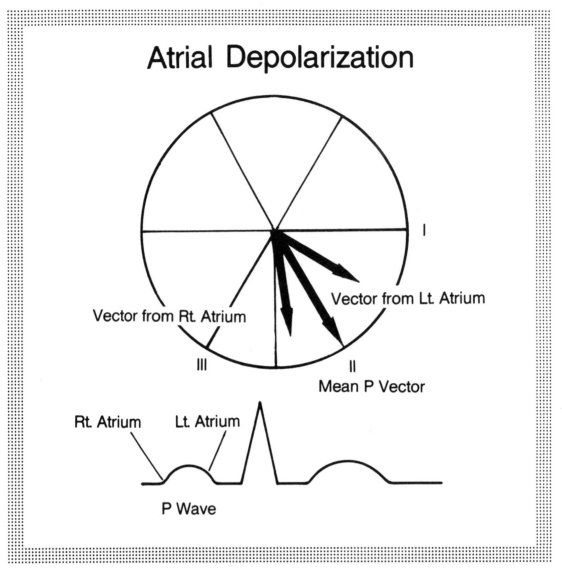

Atrial Depolarization

The mean P vector represents both atria. In order to understand atrial enlargement, we will study each atrium separately. The right atrium depolarizes first, represented by the initial portion of the P wave, followed by left atrial depolarization. The earlier right atrial vector is more rightward and anteriorly oriented compared with the left atrial vector, which is more leftward and posteriorly oriented.

In comparing right and left atrial depolarization:

right atrial depolarization occurs _____ .   earlier

the left atrial vector is oriented more _____   leftward
and _____ .   posteriorly

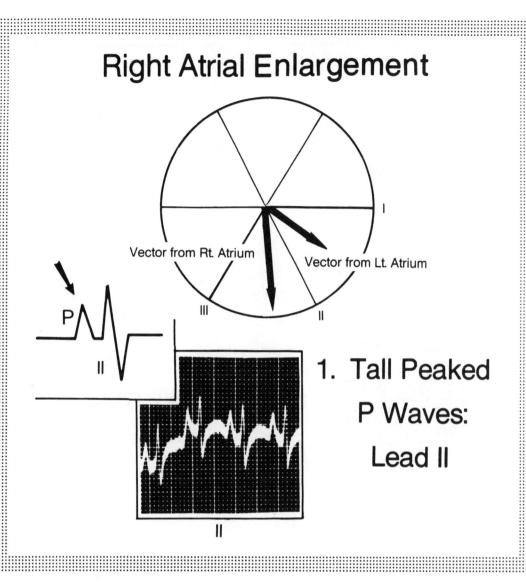

Right Atrial Enlargement

Vector from Rt. Atrium

Vector from Lt. Atrium

P

II

1. Tall Peaked P Waves: Lead II

II

In right atrial enlargement the right atrial vector, facing leads II, III, and aVF, results in *tall early P waves* in these leads. The normal P wave is rarely more than 2.5 mm. in any lead and is rounded in contour, not peaked or notched. Two common causes of right atrial enlargement are congenital heart disease and pulmonary disease. The tall peaked P wave of right atrial enlargement is frequently called "P pulmonale."

Electrocardiographic evidence of right atrial enlargement includes tall, peaked P waves in leads _____ , _____ , and _____ .

II, III
aVF

The tall, peaked P wave of right atrial hypertrophy is frequently called _____ _____ because of its association with pulmonary disease.

P pulmonale

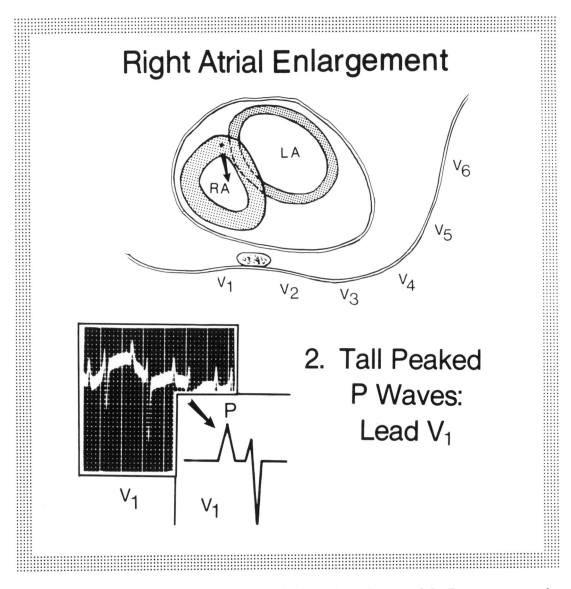

Right Atrial Enlargement

2. Tall Peaked P Waves: Lead V₁

Since the right atrial vector is *anterior,* facing lead V_1, the early part of the P wave, or even the entire P wave, may be *positive* and of great magnitude in lead V_1 in right atrial enlargement. This is in contrast to left atrial enlargement in which the orientation of the left atrial vector is *posterior,* facing away from lead V_1, with deep *negative* P waves in lead V_1 (pages 107 to 109).

The P wave is normally rarely taller than _____ mm.   **2.5**

Because the right atrial vector is anterior, the P wave in lead _____ may be positive and of great magnitude in right atrial enlargement.   **V_1**

Right Atrial Enlargement
Principal Criteria
Review

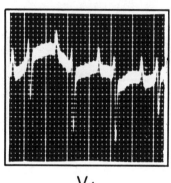

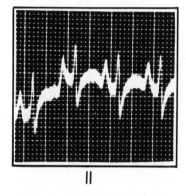

II

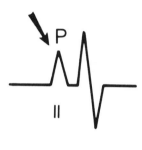

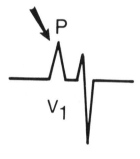

V₁

Review

In right atrial enlargement we see tall early peaked P waves in:
    Lead II, often also in leads III and aVF
    Lead V_1

Note: When evidence of right atrial enlargement is found in the electrocardiogram in the absence of tricuspid valve stenosis, it is good *presumptive evidence* of right *ventricular* hypertrophy because right atrial enlargement rarely occurs alone.

**The two most important leads in the evaluation of right atrial
enlargement are leads _____ and _____ .**   II V_1

**When evidence of right atrial enlargement is found on the
electrocardiogram in the absence of tricuspid valve stenosis, it is
good _____ evidence of right ventricular hypertrophy.**   presumptive

Left Atrial Enlargement

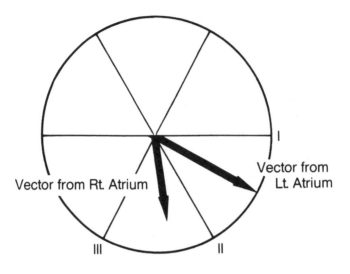

1. Broad Notched P Waves: Lead I

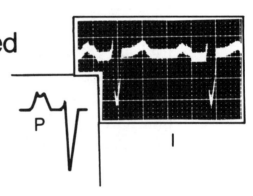

Left atrial depolarization starts after right atrial depolarization. In left atrial enlargement, the left atrial vector, facing leads I and II, is delayed with *broadening* of the latter part of the P wave, forming a *notched P wave.* Since this was commonly seen in mitral valve disease, it became known as *P mitrale.*

In left atrial enlargement, the P wave in leads I and II
is _____ and _____; it is often
called _____ _____ , because it was commonly seen in mitral
value disease.

broad notched
P mitrale

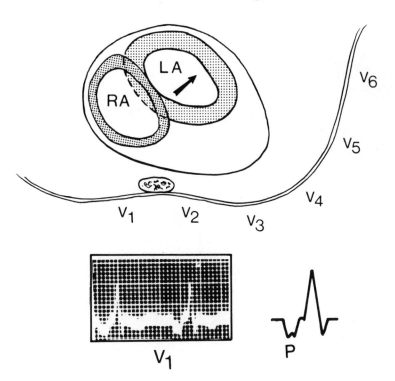

Left Atrial Enlargement

2. Negative, Notched P Waves: Lead V₁

Since the left atrial is *posterior,* facing away from lead V_1, the P wave in left atrial enlargement may be markedly *negative, broad,* and *notched.* This is in contrast to the orientation of the right atrial vector, as already noted, which is anterior, facing lead V_1, with tall positive P waves in lead V_1 in right atrial enlargement.

The left atrial vector is _____ oriented, inscribing a _____ P wave in lead V_1.

posteriorly
negative

Left Atrial Enlargement

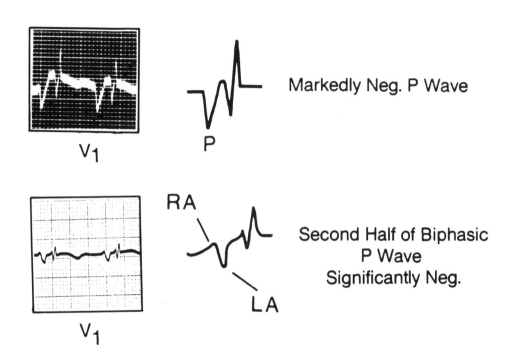

V₁

P

Markedly Neg. P Wave

RA

LA

Second Half of Biphasic
P Wave
Significantly Neg.

V₁

Additional Types of P Wave Configurations in Lead V₁

In addition to the negative, broad, and notched P wave seen on the previous page, two additional types of P waves may be seen in lead V₁ in association with left atrial enlargement. The common characteristic is that *either the entire P wave or the second part is abnormally negative.*

In left atrial enlargement, in lead V₁, the second half of a biphasic P wave may be markedly _____ .   negative

---

> Refer to page 366 for additional information on criteria for left atrial enlargement.

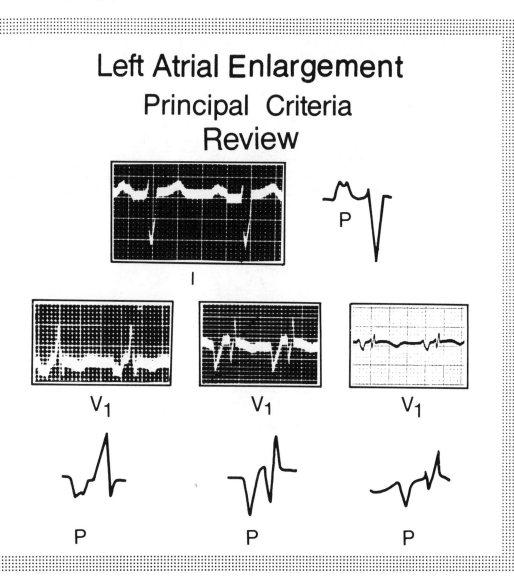

Left Atrial Enlargement
Principal Criteria
Review

Review

In left atrial enlargement the following types of P waves may be seen:

In lead I, _____ , and _____ .   broad notched

In lead V₁:

    broad, notched, and _____ .   negative

    entirely _____ .   negative

    the second half of the _____ P wave is negative.   biphasic

Biatrial Enlargement

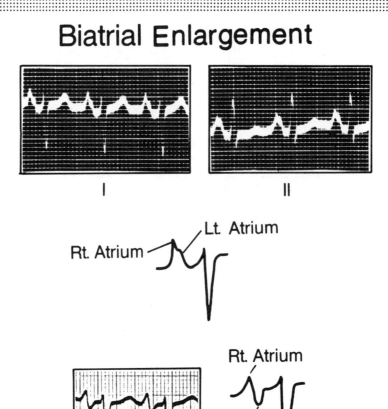

Biatrial hypertrophy has features of both right and left atrial enlargement. In leads I and II we have the early peaking of the P wave of right atrial enlargement and the notching of left atrial enlargement. In lead V_1 we see the prominent first half of the biphasic P wave of right atrial enlargement and the significantly negative second half, representing left atrial enlargement.

In biatrial enlargement:

the P waves in leads I and II display the early _____ of right atrial enlargement and the _____ of left atrial enlargement.	peaking notching
in lead V_1 the prominent first half of the biphasic P wave represents right atrial enlargement and the significantly _____ second half represents left atrial enlargement.	negative

Practice
ECG Analysis

Practice
ECG Analysis

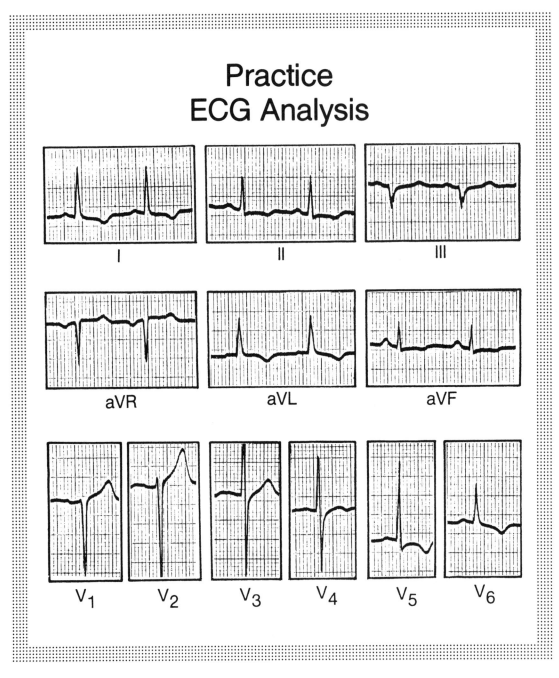

The patient is a 69-year-old woman with a history of high blood pressure.

Analysis:

ECG ANALYSIS

1. Rhythm and rate
   Rhythm: sinus
   Rate: 80/min.
   P-R interval: 0.16 sec.
2. QRS complex
   Duration: 0.08 sec.
   Axis: $+15°$
   $S_{V_2} + R_{V_5} = 45$ mm.
3. Ventricular repolarization
   S-T segment: depressed in leads II, aVF, and V_5
   T wave: T waves inverted in leads I, II, aVF, V_5, and V_6
   QRS-T angle very wide
4. Q-T interval: 0.38 sec.

Impression and Comment

Sinus rhythm
Left ventricular hypertrophy (LVH)
Ventricular repolarization (ST-T) abnormalities secondary to LVH

Increased magnitude of the ventricular deflections (QRS complexes) is the major electrocardiographic criterion for left ventricular hypertrophy, seen best in the precordial leads, V_1 to V_6. The diagnosis of left ventricular hypertrophy should not be made without evidence of increased magnitude. Ventricular repolarization (ST-T) abnormalities usually accompany left ventricular hypertrophy, although ischemia of the myocardium may additionally contribute.

Practice
ECG Analysis

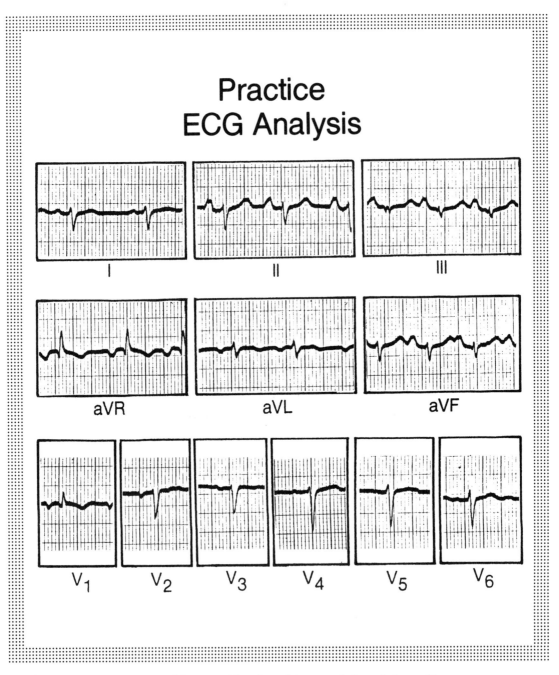

The patient is a 73-year-old man with a long history of chronic lung disease.

Analysis

ECG ANALYSIS

1. Rhythm and rate
   Rhythm: sinus
   Rate: 95/min.
   P-R interval: 0.18 sec.
   Prominent P waves, leads II, III, and aVF
2. QRS complex
   Duration: 0.08 sec.
   Axis: −120° (extreme right axis deviation)
   R wave in lead V_1 is the main ventricular deflection
3. Ventricular repolarization
   S-T segment: neither significantly elevated nor depressed
   T wave: abnormally wide QRS-T angle
4. Q-T Interval: 0.35 sec.

Impression and Comment

Sinus rhythm
Right ventricular hypertrophy (RVH)
Ventricular repolarization abnormalities secondary to RVH

The extreme right axis deviation (−135°) and the predominant R wave in lead V_1, as well as the abnormally wide QRS-T angle, are the important criteria. The prominent P waves in leads II, III, and aVF represent the accompanying right atrial hypertrophy. This patient, who had been smoking for more than 50 years, was suffering from bronchitis, emphysema, and heart failure.

Chapter 3

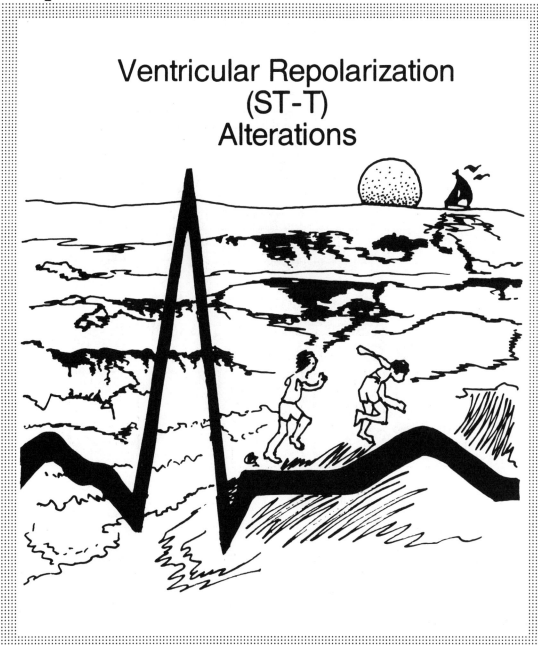

Ventricular Repolarization (ST-T) Alterations

Ventricular *repolarization* (ST-T) is a longer process and consumes more energy than *depolarization.* It is, therefore, much more prone to alterations and abnormalities; hence the multiple causes of ST-T abnormalities. On the other hand, not every S-T segment or T wave that appears abnormal at first is actually abnormal. This can be observed in the *early repolarization* and *juvenile* patterns, to be seen shortly. We have actually started studying ventricular repolarization in the first two chapters.

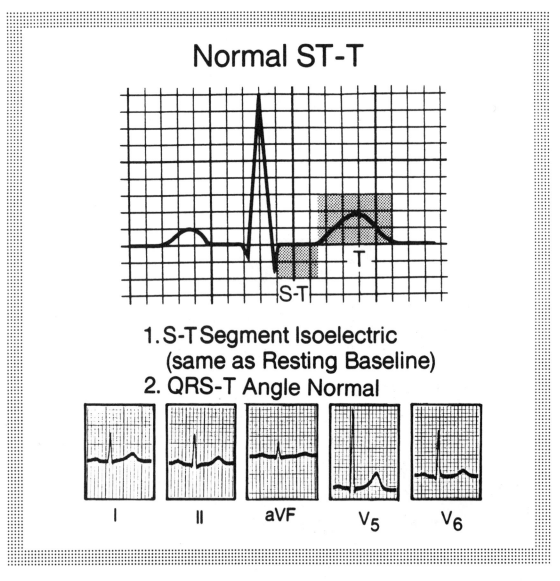

Normal ST-T

1. S-T Segment Isoelectric (same as Resting Baseline)
2. QRS-T Angle Normal

| I | II | aVF | V₅ | V₆ |

When we studied the normal adult in the first chapter, we found that often the QRS-T angle is less than 45° and rarely wider than 60°. *For the QRS-T angle to be normally narrow, the T wave should have the same orientation as the QRS complex in leads I, II, aVF, V₅, and V₆.*

The S-T segment is normally *isoelectric, the same as the resting baseline, neither elevated nor depressed.* It may, however, slope upward toward a relatively tall T wave.

The normal QRS-T angle is rarely wider than _____ .   **60°**

The normal S-T segment is _____ , the same as the resting baseline.   **isoelectric**

ST-T
Right Ventricular Hypertrophy

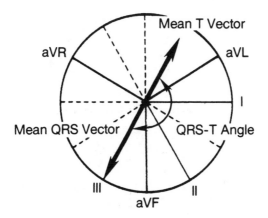

1. S-T Segment Depressed
2. QRS-T Angle Wide

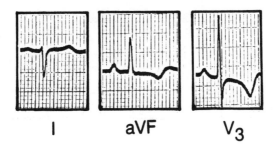

| I | aVF | V₃ |

In Chapter 2 we found that ventricular repolarization abnormalities are frequently secondary to right ventricular hypertrophy. In the above electrocardiogram, note the wide QRS-T angle. The QRS complexes and T waves are opposite in orientation. Where the QRS complex is positive, the T wave is negative, and where the QRS complex is negative, the T wave is positive. *The QRS-T angle is therefore extremely wide, 180°.* S-T segment depression is seen in lead V_3.

In the above electrocardiogram, the QRS complex is negative in lead I and positive in lead aVF,
indicating _____ _____ _____ .   right axis deviation.

The T wave is exactly opposite the QRS complex, positive in

lead I and negative in lead aVF,
indicating _____ _____ _____ .   left axis deviation

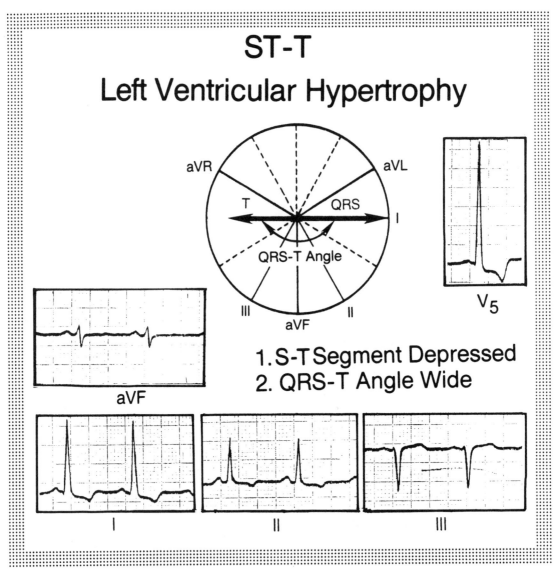

ST-T
Left Ventricular Hypertrophy

1. S-T Segment Depressed
2. QRS-T Angle Wide

As in right ventricular hypertrophy, ventricular repolarization abnormalities generally accompany left ventricular hypertrophy. Note the very wide QRS-T angle above. Where the QRS complex is positive, the T wave is negative, and where the QRS complex is negative, the T wave is positive. They share the transition at lead aVF. S-T segment depression is seen in leads I and V₅.

In this electrocardiogram, the QRS complex and T wave are transitional in lead _____ .

aVF

The QRS-T angle is _____ .

180°

ST-T
Bundle Branch Block

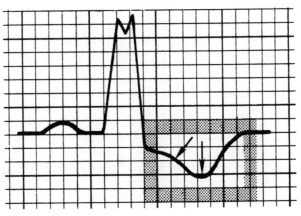

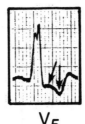

V₅

1. S-T Segment Depressed
2. QRS-T Angle Wide

This electrocardiogram represents an intraventricular conduction disturbance (left bundle branch block), studied in Chapter 5. For the present, note the abnormal width of the QRS complex and the repolarization abnormalities. When depolarization is abnormal, as seen above, repolarization is secondarily also abnormal.

When ventricular depolarization is prolonged, as in an intraventricular conduction disturbance,

_____ **is secondarily also abnormal.**   repolarization

The S-T segment may be _____ and the QRS-T   depressed
angle _____ .   widened

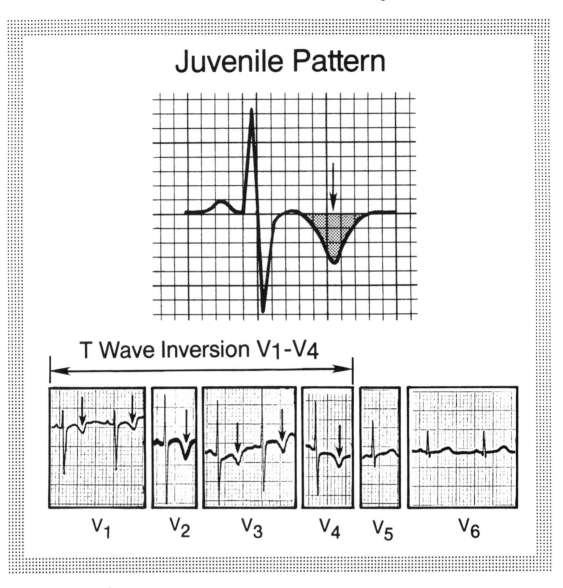

In youth the mean T vector is frequently to the left, inferior, and posterior, inscribing T waves across the chest that are negative in leads V_1, V_2, V_3, and often V_4. This is known as the *juvenile pattern*. This pattern is not infrequently seen in normal healthy young patients well into the third decade of life. This emphasizes that the electrocardiogram should not be read without knowing the age of the patient or without knowledge of the clinical history.[5,6]

The finding of negative T waves across the chest in leads V_1, V_2, V_3, and often V_4 in a healthy young patient is known as the _____ _____ .   juvenile pattern

The importance of knowing the _____ and   age
clinical _____ is emphasized in electrocardiographic   history
interpretation.

Digitalis Effects

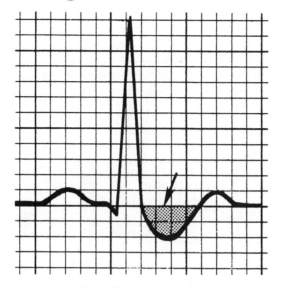

S-T Segment Sloping Downward

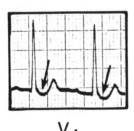

V$_4$

Digitalis has long been known for its effects on the entire phase of ventricular repolarization, both the S-T segment and the T wave, depressing the S-T segment and widening the QRS-T angle. The "classic" changes of digitalis, however, refer to the effects on the S-T segment, often described as a *paintbrush inscription* (as if you were painting the S-T segment with gradual widening of the brush stroke), or a *fist-like depression* of the S-T segment (as if you were placing a fist in the S-T segment and depressing it), or *scooping* of the S-T segment.

Digitalis effects on the S-T segment have been variously described as   paintbrush
a _____ inscription, _____   fist-like
depression, and _____ .   scooping

Early Repolarization

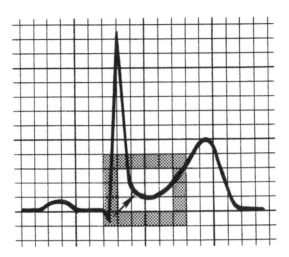

Elevated "Takeoff" of S-T Segment

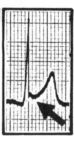

V_3

A common repolarization variant, seen in normal young adults, is S-T segment displacement, usually associated with tall or deep T waves.[7,8] This pattern has been known as *early repolarization* and is not considered abnormal. Note the elevation of the QRS-ST junction (J point). The electrocardiogram is normal in all other aspects. Of importance is the need to distinguish early repolarization from the more ominous causes of S-T segment displacement, such as pericarditis and myocardial infarction.

Early repolarization:

is considered a _____ repolarization variant.   **normal**

is usually associated with _____ or _____ T waves.   **tall deep**

Pericarditis

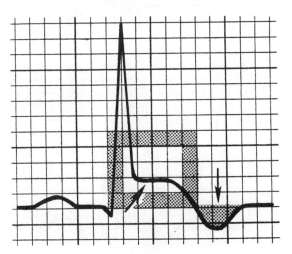

1. S-T Segment Elevated
2. T Wave Inverted

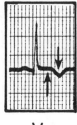

V₆

Ventricular repolarization abnormalities are common in patients with acute *pericarditis.*[9-11] Often both the S-T segment and the T wave are involved. Do not confuse this abnormal, changing, and evolving pattern with early repolarization found in healthy young patients. Clinical correlation must be stressed, since the electrocardiographic changes seen above may not be distinguishable from those of a patient with an acute myocardial infarction.

In early repolarization the electrocardiographic pattern is stable, whereas in acute pericarditis the pattern is constantly _____ .

changing

The electrocardiographic changes in acute pericarditis may not be distinguishable from those of a patient with a (an) _____ _____ .

myocardial infarction

Coronary Heart Disease with Exercise

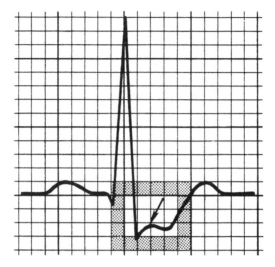

S-T Segment Depression

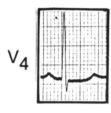

V_4

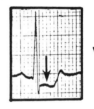

V_4

Baseline   Exercise

Coronary heart disease is a major cause of *primary* ventricular repolarization abnormalities. It is *primary* because it is a problem within the phase of repolarization and not *secondary* to an abnormality in depolarization as occurs in bundle branch block (page 121) or *secondary* to ventricular hypertrophy (pages 119 and 120). A patient with secondary repolarization abnormalities may also have additional primary abnormalities. In the above recording, the marked depression with exercise of the S-T segment occurred in a patient with a history of angina pectoris. Some patients with a typical history of angina pectoris have an electrocardiogram with normal ventricular repolarization *at rest* that becomes abnormal during a graded stress test.[12] Often, utilizing the patient's normal activity, such as taking a walk, yields important information in the initial evaluation.

_____ _____ _____ is a major   **Coronary heart disease**
cause of ventricular repolarization abnormalities.

_____ _____ often reveals ventricular   **Stress testing**
repolarization abnormalities not seen on the resting
electrocardiogram.

Coronary Heart Disease
Angina Pectoris

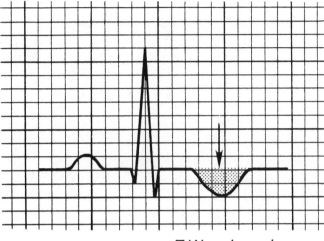

T Wave Inversion

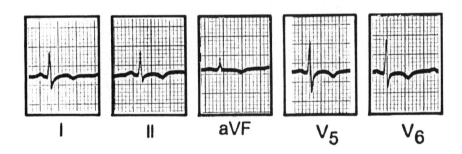

| I | II | aVF | V$_5$ | V$_6$ |

A wide QRS-T angle is often found in coronary heart disease patients with angina pectoris. Note that the QRS complexes and T waves are opposite in orientation. The term *ischemia* is frequently applied to this wide QRS-T angle. When the cause is not known, this abnormality often is labeled *nonspecific*. (Refer to page 361 for discussion of sensitivity and specificity).

A _____ QRS-T angle is commonly found in patients with coronary heart disease.   wide

Ventricular repolarization abnormalities, when the cause is not known, are often labeled _____ .   nonspecific

Variant Angina Pectoris
(Angina Pectoris at Rest)

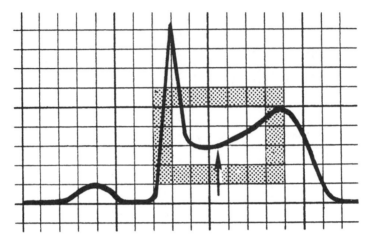

S-T Segment Elevated

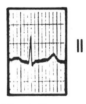   II

Baseline

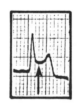   II

During Pain

A variant form of angina pectoris was reported by Prinzmetal.[13,14] The striking elevation of the S-T segment in lead II occurred in a patient with a history of angina pectoris, principally *at rest*. This marked S-T segment elevation resembles that of the hyperacute phase of myocardial infarction (next chapter) but lasts only a few minutes. This disorder is commonly caused by spasm of the coronary arteries.

Prinzmetal's angina:
is a variant form of angina, occurring principally _____ _____ .   at rest

is commonly caused by _____ of the coronary arteries.   spasm

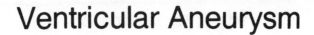

Ventricular Aneurysm

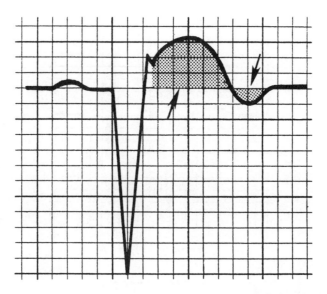

1. S-T Segment Elevated
2. T Wave Inverted

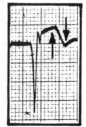

V₂

The persistent elevation of the S-T segment, described as a *monophasic curve of injury,* represents a ventricular aneurysm, an outpouching of a section of scarred ventricular myocardium. The electrocardiogram resembles that of an acute myocardial infarction (next chapter). In order to exclude an acute myocardial infarction, always ask for comparison electrocardiograms.

A ventricular aneurysm may resemble electrocardiographically an acute _____ _____ .

myocardial infarction

Comparison electrocardiograms

_____ _____ help one to differentiate a ventricular aneurysm from an acute myocardial infarction.

Hypokalemia

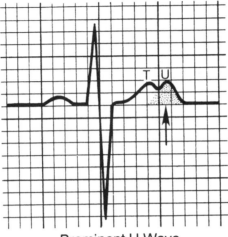

Prominent U Wave

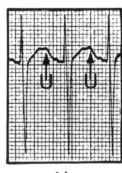

V₂

Hypokalemia (low potassium level) may produce striking electrocardiographic abnormalities, such as depression of the S-T segment, lowering and flattening of the T wave, and appearance of a *U wave*. The U wave is a wave that follows the T wave and has frequently been associated with hypokalemia, although it may be found normally. During correction of the hypokalemia, close electrocardiographic follow-up of this patient revealed a T wave that gradually became taller and a U wave that gradually disappeared.

The electrocardiographic manifestations of hypokalemia include _____ _____ , _____ _____ _____ , and appearance of a _____ _____ .

S-T depression
lowered T wave
U wave

> See page 367 for further elaboration on this patient.

U Wave

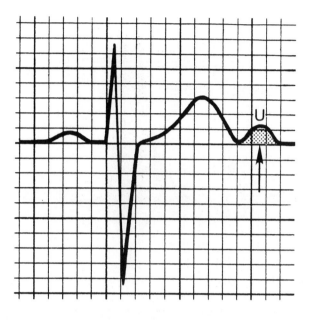

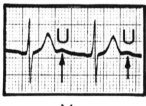

V_4

Although the U wave, which follows the T wave, has been associated with hypokalemia (which causes its accentuation), it may be found normally. It is often seen best in the midprecordial leads (V_3 and V_4, as above), and it has the same orientation as the T wave. When it is found normally in these leads, it is a *positive* U wave. A negative U wave has been associated with systemic hypertension, aortic and mitral regurgitation, and ischemic heart disease.[15,16]

When the U wave is found normally, it is best seen in leads _____ and _____ .

V_3
V_4

A _____ U wave has been associated with various heart disorders.

negative

Hyperkalemia

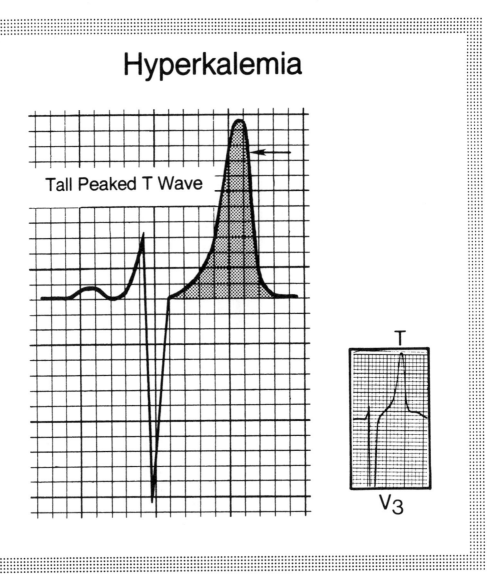

Tall Peaked T Wave

The appearance of *a tall, peaked T wave* is a manifestation of hyperkalemia (high potassium level). With increasingly high blood levels of potassium, the P-R interval is prolonged, with a widening QRS interval. In more extreme cases of hyperkalemia, the P waves become flatter and the QRS complexes continue to widen. Ventricular fibrillation may then ensue if the level of potassium continues to rise.

**The electrocardiographic manifestations of hyperkalemia include a
peaked _____ _____ , prolongation of the _____ interval, and
a _____ QRS complex.**

T wave, P-R
widening

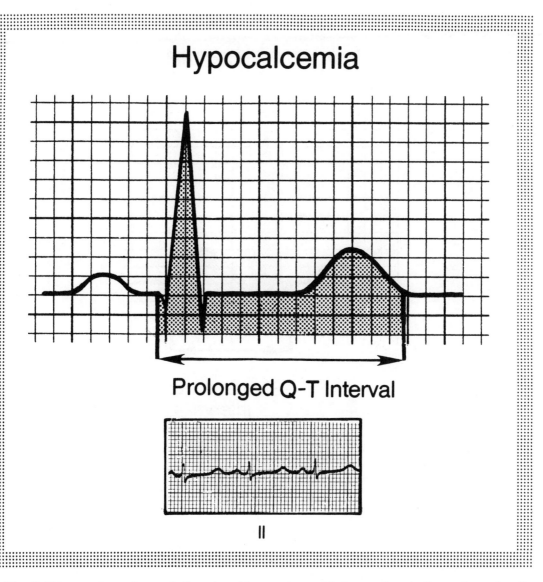

Hypocalcemia

Prolonged Q-T Interval

II

The Q-T interval may be *markedly prolonged* in a patient with hypocalcemia (low calcium level). This patient's heart rate is 84 per min. At this rate the Q-T interval should be approximately 0.35 sec. rather than 0.52 sec., as seen here. Review page 66 (relationship between the Q-T interval and the heart rate).

Review

The normal Q-T interval at a rate of 84 is approximately _____ sec.   0.35

Electrocardiographic evidence of hypocalcemia may be a
marked _____ of the Q-T interval.   prolongation

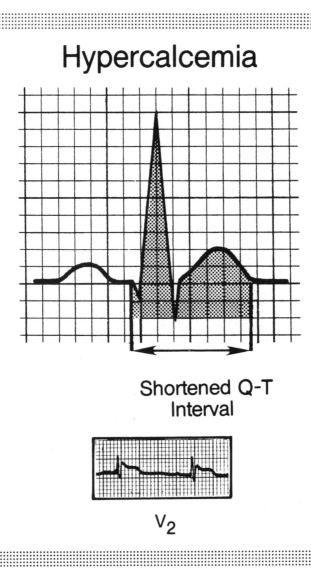

Hypercalcemia

Shortened Q-T
Interval

V_2

Hypercalcemia (high calcium level) is often represented electrocardiographically by a *short Q-T interval.* There is an inverse relationship between the Q-T interval and the level of serum calcium. The P-R interval may also be prolonged.

A _____ Q-T interval may be an electrocardiographic   short
manifestation of hypercalcemia.

The _____ interval may also be prolonged.   P-R

Practice
ECG Analysis

Practice
ECG Analysis

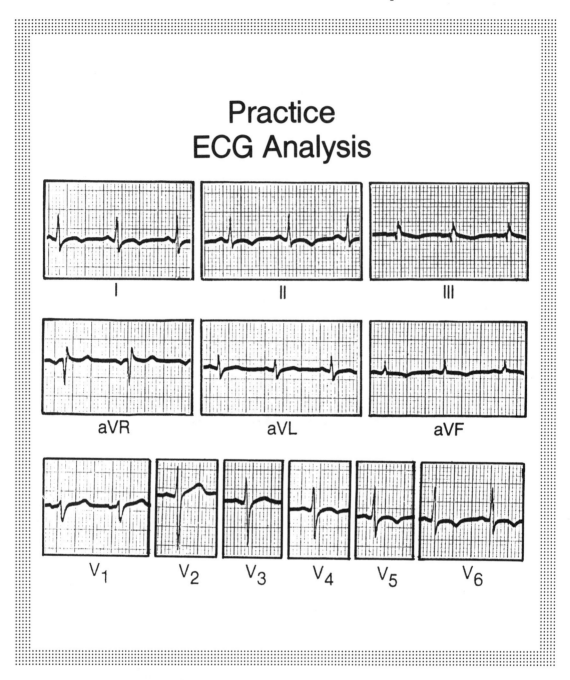

The patient is a 60 year old man with a history of stable angina pectoris, responsive to treatment with nitroglycerin.

Analysis:

ECG ANALYSIS

1. Rhythm and rate
   Rhythm: sinus
   Rate: 90/min.
   P-R interval: 0.14 sec.
2. QRS complex
   Duration: 0.08 sec.
   Axis: $+60°$
3. Ventricular repolarization
   S-T segment: not significantly elevated or depressed
   T wave: inverted in leads I, II, III, aVF, and V_4 to V_6; QRS-T angle very wide
4. Q-T interval: 0.36 sec.

Impression and Comment

Sinus rhythm
Ventricular repolarization abnormalities compatible with coronary heart disease

A wide QRS-T angle is frequently found in coronary heart disease patients with angina pectoris. Note that the QRS complexes and T waves are opposite in orientation. The term *ischemia* is often applied to this wide QRS-T angle. Evaluation of this patient revealed significant coronary heart disease with myocardial ischemia.

Practice
ECG Analysis

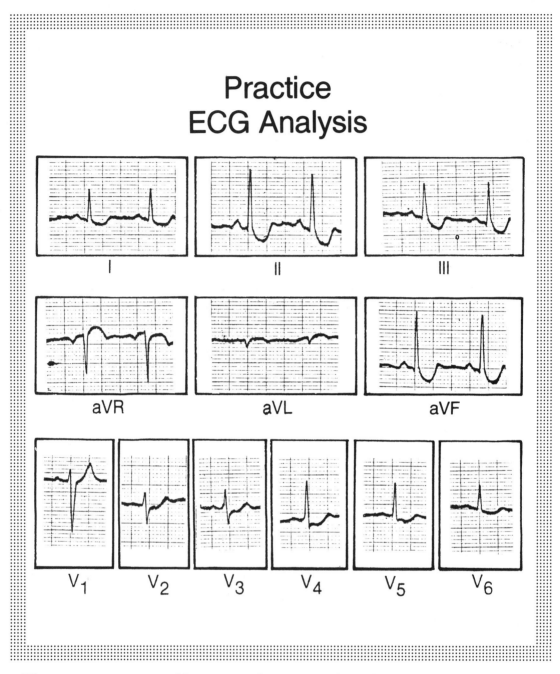

The patient is a 75-year-old woman with congestive heart failure, for which she is taking digitalis and diuretics.

Analysis:

ECG ANALYSIS

1. Rhythm and rate
   Rhythm: sinus
   Rate: 85 min.
   P-R interval: 0.16 sec.
2. QRS complex
   Duration: 0.08 sec.
   Axis: + 65°
3. Ventricular repolarization
   S-T segment: rounded S-T segments, depressed in leads I, II, III, aVF, and V_6, elevated in lead aVR; S-T segment also depressed in leads V_2 to V_5
   T wave: flat or low in leads I, II, III, aVF, V_5, and V_6, inverted in aVL; however, the QRS-T angle is not wide
4. Q-T interval: 0.34 sec.

Impression and Comment

Sinus rhythm
Ventricular repolarization alterations compatible with digitalis effects and myocardial ischemia

The paintbrush inscription of the S-T segments, seen especially well in leads II, III, and aVF, as well as the lowering and flattening of the T waves, is commonly seen as a result of "digitalis effects." The depressed origin or "take-off" of the S-T segments (J point) in leads V_2, V_3, V_4, and V_5, present before the patient started taking digitalis, is compatible with the myocardial ischemia from her known coronary heart disease.

Chapter 4

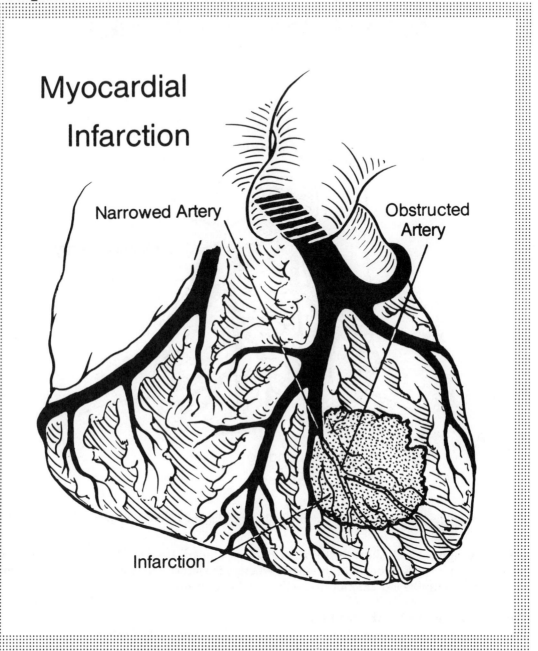

Myocardial Infarction

Narrowed Artery

Obstructed Artery

Infarction

When the blood supply to an area of the heart is obstructed, a section of heart muscle may die. This is known as infarction of the heart muscle or *myocardial infarction.*

Normal Coronary Arteries

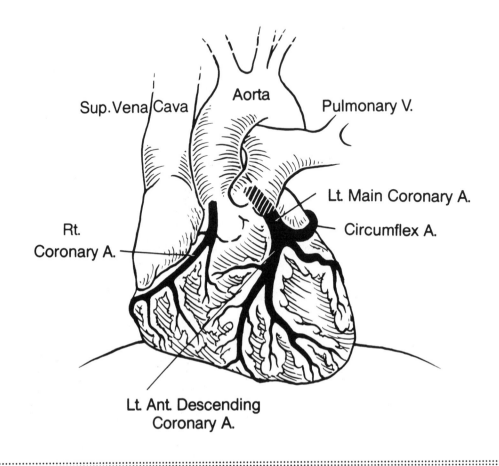

Blood is supplied to the heart by the right and left coronary arteries. The right coronary artery remains a major trunk throughout its length, whereas the left coronary artery, after a short main stem, divides into the left anterior descending and circumflex arteries.

The heart is supplied with blood through the _____ _____ .	coronary arteries
The left coronary artery after, a short main stem, divides into the _____ _____ _____ **and** _____ **arteries.**	left anterior descending circumflex

Left Ventricle

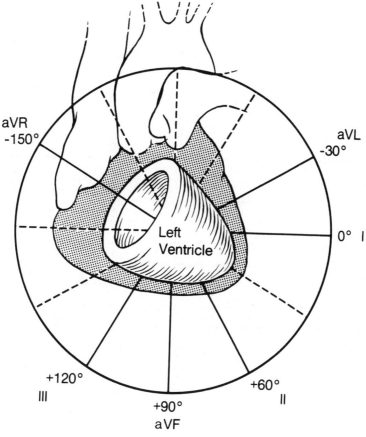

The left ventricle is the chamber of the heart most frequently associated with myocardial infarction. Although the left ventricle is the subject of this chapter, myocardial infarction of the right ventricle is also illustrated (page 368).

Myocardial infarction:

most frequently involves the _____ **ventricle.**   **left**

may also involve the _____ **ventricle.**   **right**

> Right ventricular infarction is illustrated on page 368.

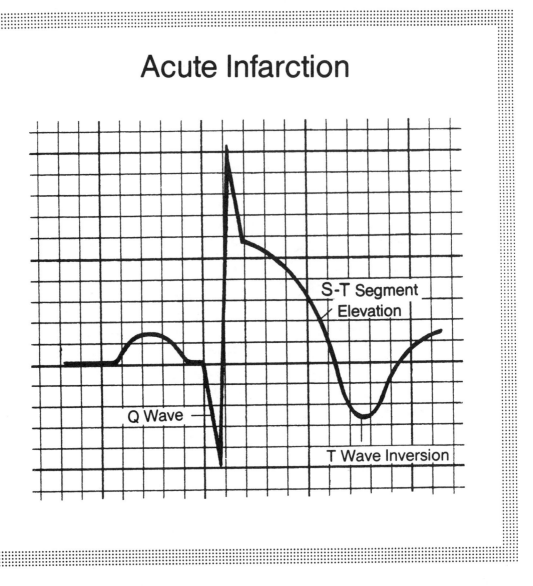

The classic electrocardiographic changes encountered in acute myocardial infarction are:

1. _____   **The Q wave**
2. _____   **S-T segment elevation**
3. _____   **T wave inversion**

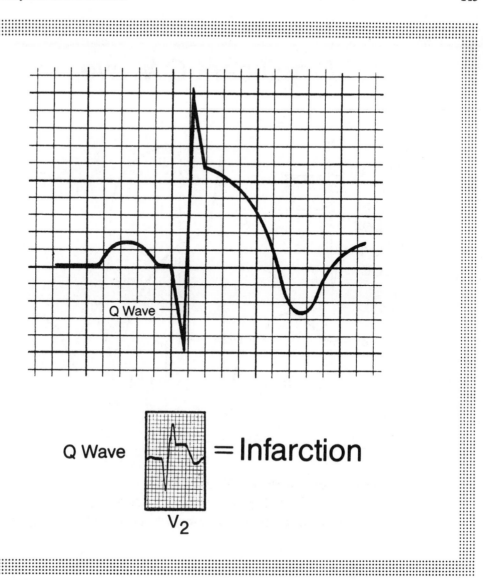

Q Wave = Infarction

V_2

The Q wave is *the electrocardiographic manifestation of myocardial infarction.* The Q wave must, however, be *significant,* since in normal patients small Q waves are frequently seen in various leads (I, aVL, V_5, V_6). The significant Q wave is illustrated on the next page.

The _____ _____ is the electrocardiographic manifestation of myocardial infarction.

Q wave

In leads I and V_6, a small Q wave is _____ .

normal

Significant Q Wave

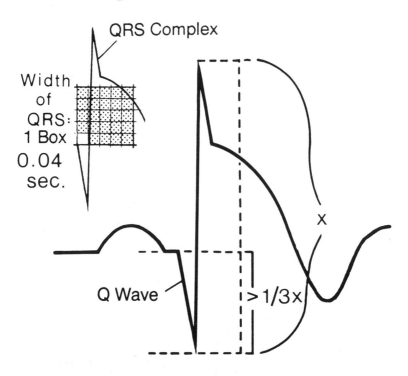

A significant Q wave should be:
1. One-third height of QRS complex
2. 0.04 second (one small box wide) in duration

The *significant Q wave* is at least *one third the height of the QRS complex* and *0.04 sec. in duration (one small box wide).* Lead aVR is the exception, since a large Q wave may be seen normally.

The significant Q wave is at least:
1. _____   **one third the height of the QRS complex**
2. _____   **0.04 sec. in duration**

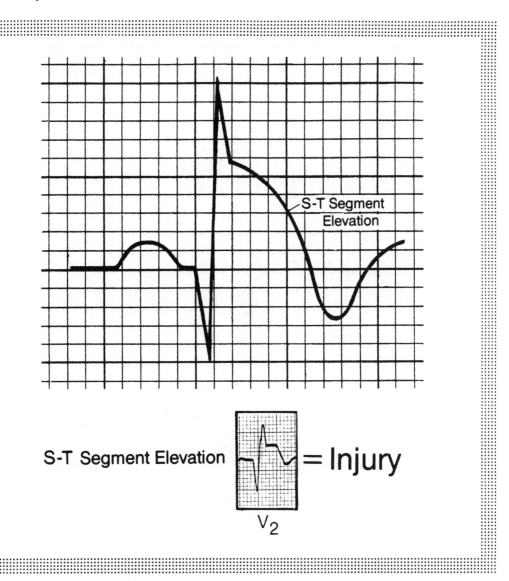

S-T Segment Elevation = Injury

V_2

The elevated S-T segment seen in acute myocardial infarction is known as the *current of injury*. Because of its appearance, it is sometimes referred to as the *monophasic curve of injury*.

In acute myocardial infarction the elevated S-T segment represents _____ **; it is sometimes called the** _____ **curve of injury.**

injury

monophasic

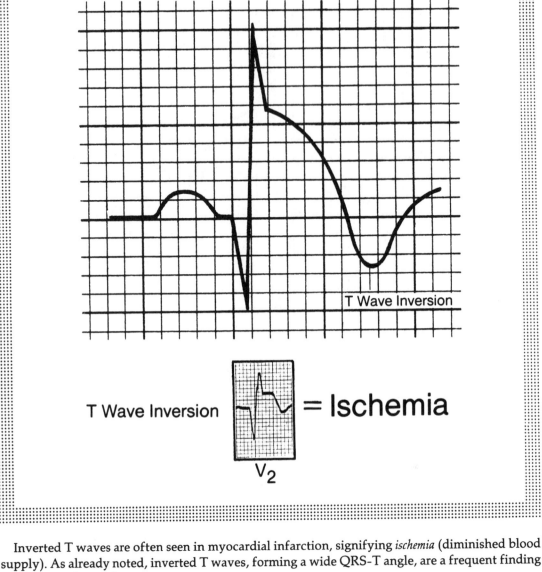

Inverted T waves are often seen in myocardial infarction, signifying *ischemia* (diminished blood supply). As already noted, inverted T waves, forming a wide QRS-T angle, are a frequent finding in electrocardiography.

In acute myocardial infarction:
the inverted T wave represents _____ .   ischemia

a _____ QRS-T angle is commonly seen.   wide

Classic Myocardial Infarction

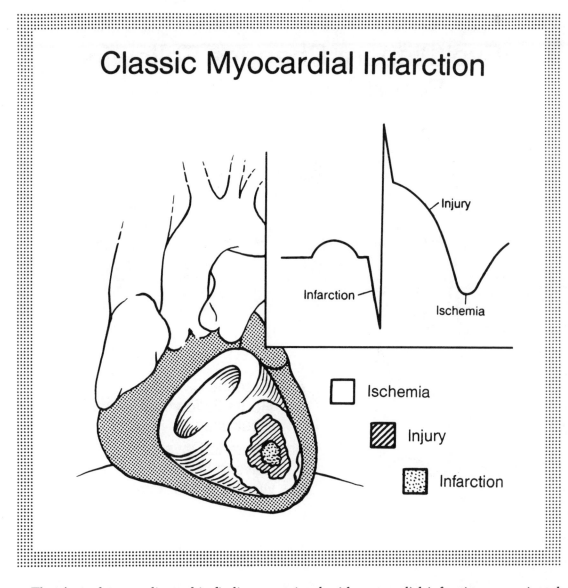

The *classic* electrocardiographic findings associated with myocardial infarction are reviewed above. Any of the three, however, may be found alone. The accompanying diagram shows an infarcted zone surrounded by zones of injury and ischemia.

To summarize, the classic electrocardiographic findings associated with acute myocardial infarction include:

1. _____
2. _____
3. _____

T wave inversion—ischemia
S-T segment elevation—injury
Q wave—infarction

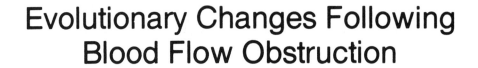

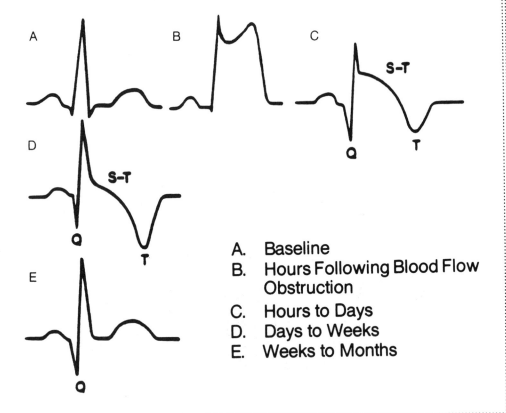

Note that the S-T segment elevation occurs prior to the formation of the Q wave. During these early hours, interventions are often undertaken to reverse the process. As time passes, the Q wave forms, the S-T segment is less elevated, and the T wave inverts. The final outcome varies greatly, depending on the amount of myocardial damage.

The evolutionary electrocardiographic changes
following blood flow obstruction to the myocardium
may be classified as follows:

1. _____   Hours following obstruction
2. _____   Hours to days
3. _____   Days to weeks
4. _____   Weeks to months

Areas of Infarction
(Left Ventricle)

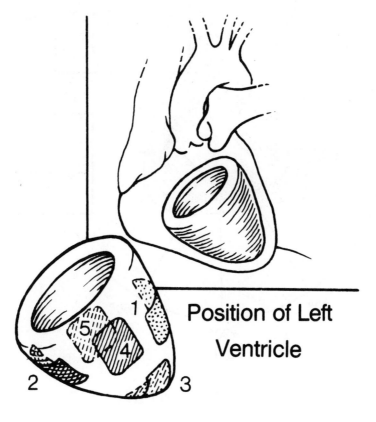

Position of Left
Ventricle

The illustration shows the division of the left ventricle into regions where infarction may occur.

These regions are:

1. _____	**Lateral**
2. _____	**Diaphragmatic or inferior**
3. _____	**Apical**
4. _____	**Anterior**
5. _____	**Posterior**

Lateral Infarction

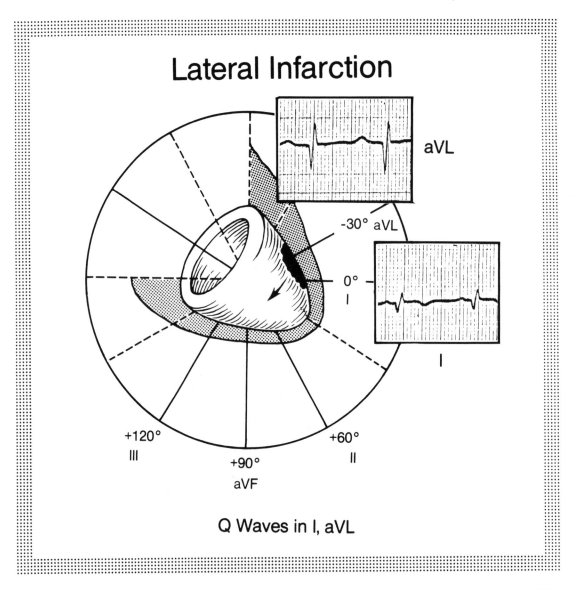

aVL

-30° aVL

0°
I

I

+120°
III

+90°
aVF

+60°
II

Q Waves in I, aVL

In *lateral* myocardial infarction, the initial vector of ventricular depolarization, the initial QRS vector (arrow), moves *away* from the lateral area, hence the formation of significant Q waves in these leads. *The Q wave represents initial vectorial forces moving away from the electrode at the point of recording.*

In lateral myocardial infarction, the initial QRS vector moves away from leads _____ and _____ , hence the formation of _____ _____ in these leads.

I aVL

Q waves

Lateral Infarction

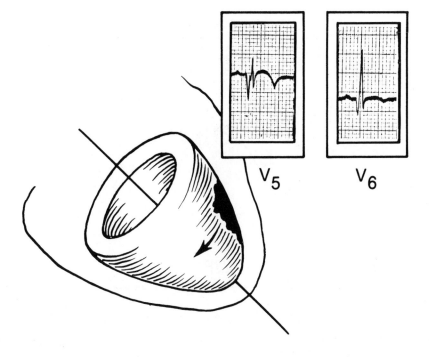

Q Waves in V5, V6

Lateral myocardial infarction may also be seen electrocardiographically with significant Q waves in the lateral precordial leads, with the initial QRS vector (arrow) moving away from these leads.

In lateral myocardial infarction, Q waves may also be seen in
leads _____ and _____, which are the V_5 V_6
_____ precordial leads.   lateral

Inferior (Diaphragmatic) Infarction

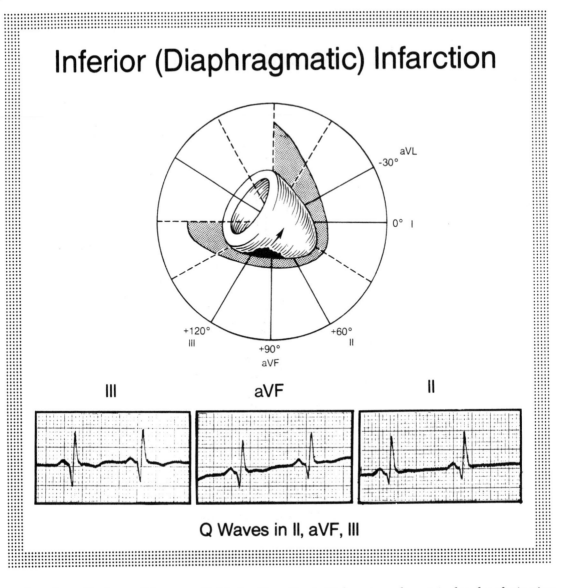

Q Waves in II, aVF, III

In *inferior (diaphragmatic)* myocardial infarction, the initial vector of ventricular depolarization moves away from the diaphragmatic area. Significant Q waves are thereby formed in these leads.

In inferior myocardial infarction, significant Q waves may be seen in the inferior leads _____ _____ and _____   II III aVF

> See page 369 for explanation and illustration of "reciprocal changes."

Apical Infarction

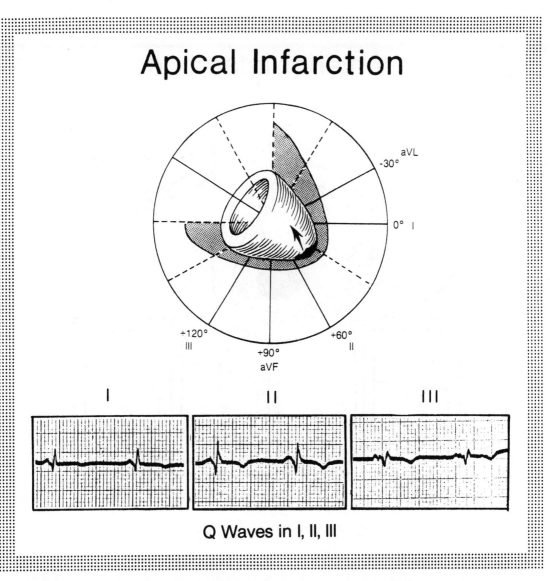

Q Waves in I, II, III

In *apical* myocardial infarction, the initial QRS vector, pointing away from the apical myocardium and from leads I, II, and III, produces Q waves in all three leads. The question arises: Did one myocardial infarction produce these abnormalities, or are they the result of the occurrence of more than one infarction at different times? Serial electrocardiograms are vital in this determination.

When significant Q waves are present in leads I, II, and III, they may
represent a(n) _____ myocardial infarction or a combination   apical
of _____ and _____ myocardial   lateral
infarctions, emphasizing the need for serial electrocardiograms.   inferior

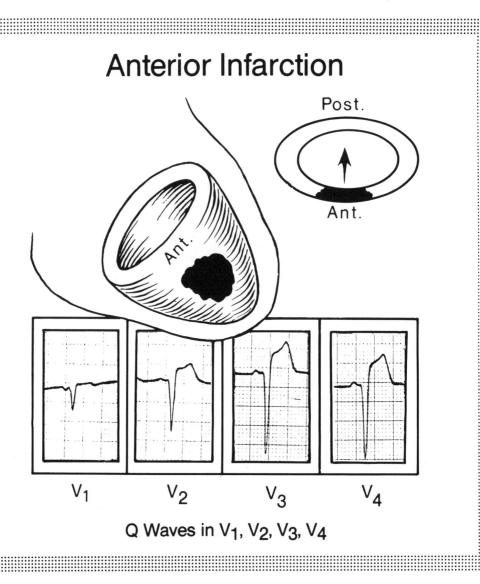

Anterior Infarction

Q Waves in V₁, V₂, V₃, V₄

In *anterior* or *anteroseptal* myocardial infarction, the initial QRS vector (arrow) moves away from the anterior surface and away from the anterior chest leads; hence the occurrence of significant Q waves in these leads. When the Q waves are limited to leads V_1 to V_3, the infarction is labeled "anteroseptal." The right-sided chest leads normally do not have Q waves of any size.

A Q wave is not _____ in the right-sided chest leads.   normal

An anteroseptal myocardial infarction may be represented
electrocardiographically by Q waves in leads _____ _____ . V_1 to V_3

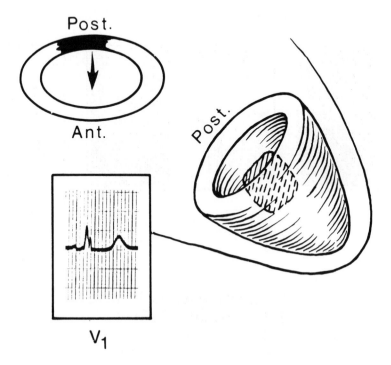

Posterior Infarction

Post.

Ant.

Post.

V_1

Prominent or Predominant R Wave in V_1

In *posterior* (often called "true posterior") myocardial infarction, the initial QRS vector (arrow) moves away from the posterior wall of the left ventricle, located posteriorly and to the left. This initial vector therefore moves anteriorly and to the right, toward lead V_1, inscribing a positive deflection, *a predominant R wave in lead V_1*. This R wave in posterior myocardial infarction represents the same phenomenon as the Q wave in anterior myocardial infarction. The prominent R wave in lead V_1 may also represent right ventricular hypertrophy (RVH, Chapter 2), right bundle branch block (RBBB), and Wolff-Parkinson-White (W-P-W) syndrome. The last two conditions will be studied shortly.

A prominent or predominant R wave in lead V_1 may represent:

1. _____   **Posterior myocardial infarction**
2. _____   **RVH**
3. _____   **RBBB**
4. _____   **W-P-W syndrome**

Infarction Without Q Waves

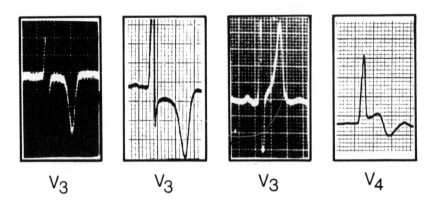

V₃   V₃   V₃   V₄

1. Deeply Inverted T Waves
2. Tall Peaked T Waves
3. S-T Segment Depressed
4. S-T Segment Elevated

Clinical evidence of infarction of the heart is frequently encountered without Q waves on the electrocardiogram. Although it may be misleading, the term *subendocardial* infarction has often been used in this context. The clinical picture of infarction should be quite clear before an electrocardiogram is labeled subendocardial infarction, since these repolarization abnormalities, although striking, may be nonspecific. Similar findings may occur during angina pectoris (negative T waves) and electrolyte imbalance (tall, peaked T waves).

Myocardial infarction without Q waves may be manifest electrocardiographically by:

1. _____   Deeply inverted T waves
2. _____   Tall, peaked T waves
3. _____   S-T segment depression
4. _____   S-T segment elevation

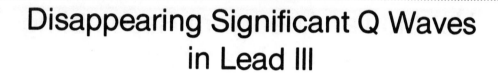

Disappearing Significant Q Waves in Lead III

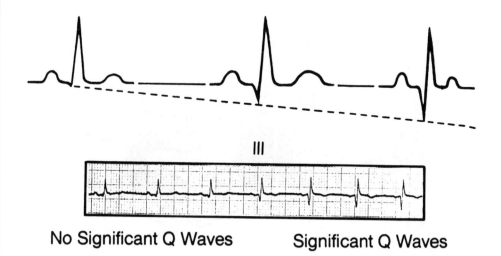

III

No Significant Q Waves   Significant Q Waves

> Disappearing significant Q waves in lead III during normal respiration may not signify myocardial infarction.

Not all Q waves signify infarction of the heart, even if they are *significant*. A Q wave in lead III may vary in size with respiration in a normal person because of slight vectorial shifts during respiration. Conversely, this *does not* mean that a Q wave in lead III may not be the result of a myocardial infarction. It is more likely to represent myocardial infarction if it is associated with Q waves in leads II and aVF. Serial electrocardiograms are helpful in providing the answer.

A Q wave in lead _____ , varying with respiration, may not signify   **III**
myocardial infarction.

This Q wave is due to _____ shifts during respiration.   **vectorial**

> Formation of the normal Q wave in lead III is illustrated on page 370.

Ventricular Aneurysm Resembling Acute Infarction

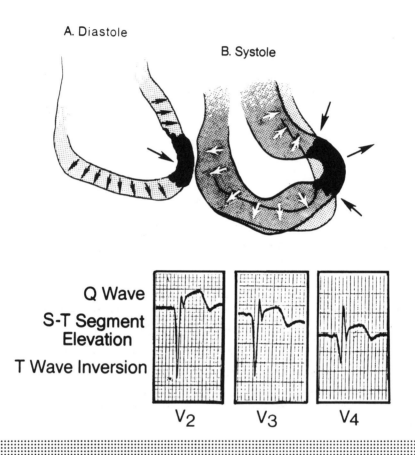

A. Diastole

B. Systole

Q Wave

S-T Segment Elevation

T Wave Inversion

V₂   V₃   V₄

This electrocardiogram, with Q waves, elevated S-T segments, and inverted T waves, could be mistaken for a representation of an acute myocardial infarction. Actually, it is from a patient with a *ventricular aneurysm,* following a myocardial infarction that occurred years earlier. A ventricular aneurysm is an outpouching (during systole, B above) of a section of scarred ventricular myocardium in systole and diastole. In order to exclude an acute myocardial infarction, always ask for comparison electrocardiograms.

The electrocardiographic pattern of an acute myocardial infarction may also represent a(n) _____ _____ , which is an outpouching of a section of scarred myocardium during _____ and _____ .

ventricular
aneurysm
systole, diastole

Practice
ECG Analysis

Practice
ECG Analysis

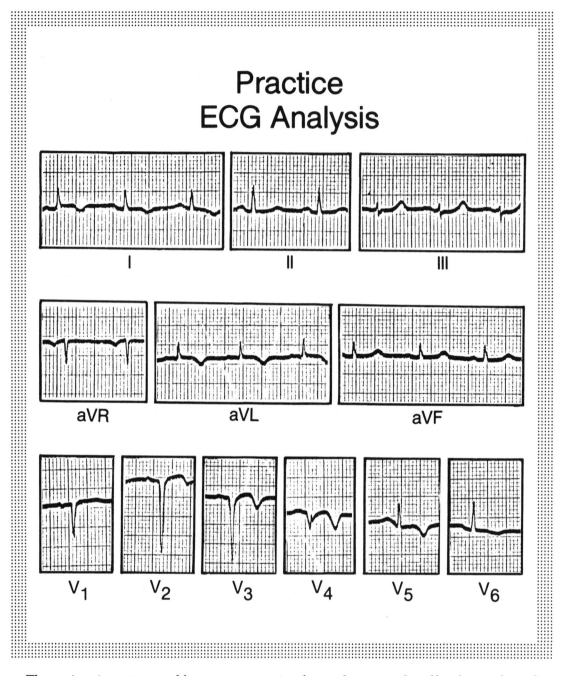

The patient is a 67-year-old woman recovering from a heart attack suffered 3 weeks earlier.

Analysis:

ECG ANALYSIS

1. Rhythm and rate
   Rhythm: sinus
   Rate: 85/min.
   P-R Interval: 0.16 sec.
2. QRS complex
   Duration: 0.08 sec.
   Axis: $+30°$
   QS complexes, leads V_1 to V_4
3. Ventricular repolarization
   S-T segment: elevated in leads V_2 and V_3
   T wave: inverted in leads 1, aVL, and V_2 to V_6; QRS-T angle wide
4. Q-T interval: 0.36 sec.

Impression and Comment

Sinus rhythm
Anterior myocardial infarction, recent
Evolving ventricular repolarization (ST-T) abnormalities, following myocardial infarction

The rounded and/or elevated S-T segments seen in leads V_2, V_3, and V_4 followed by the inverted T waves are evolutionary changes following a recent myocardial infarction. The classic electrocardiographic findings in myocardial infarction are seen here.

1. The Q wave = infarct
2. S-T segment elevation = injury
3. T wave inversion = ischemia

Practice
ECG Analysis

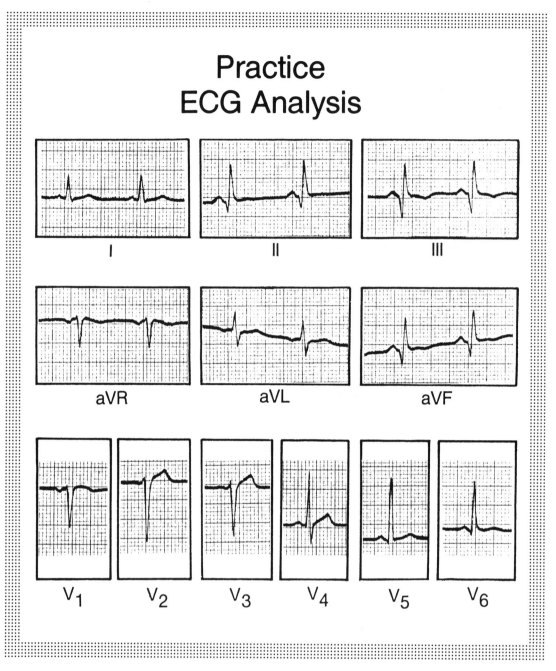

The patient is a 71-year-old woman with a history of a heart attack 3 years earlier. She becomes short of breath on moderate exertion.

Analysis:

ECG ANALYSIS

1. Rhythm and rate
   Rhythm: sinus
   Rate: 78/min.
      P-R interval: 0.14 sec.
2. QRS complex
   Duration: 0.09 sec.
   Axis: $+60°$
   Significant Q waves, leads II, III, and aVF
3. Ventricular repolarization
   S-T segment: neither significantly elevated nor depressed
   T Wave: low, but positive in leads I, aVL, V_5 and V_6, flat or transitional in lead II; QRS-T angle wide
4. Q-T Interval: 0.32 sec.

Impression and Comment

Sinus rhythm
Inferior (diaphragmatic) myocardial infarction, old
Ventricular repolarization abnormalities

This elderly patient, who had a normal electrocardiogram prior to the myocardial infarction, was left with a compromised coronary circulation as a result of the infarction. Evaluation revealed substantial coronary heart disease.

Chapter 5

Conduction Disturbances

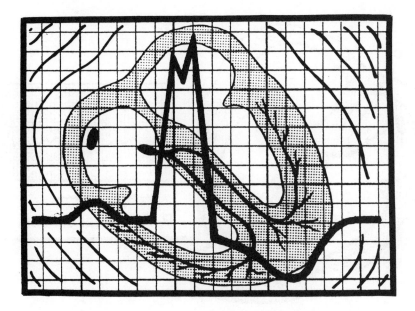

1. Atrioventricular (A-V) Conduction Disturbances

2. Intraventricular (I-V) Conduction Disturbances

As noted earlier, the heart possesses its own *specialized conduction system.* The impulse originates in the sinoatrial (S-A) node and spreads through the atria. The excitation then reaches the atrioventricular (A-V) node, located in the right atrium near the tricuspid valve. Conduction proceeds to the bundle of His, then to the left and right bundle branches (LBB and RBB). The impulse then enters the Purkinje system, and ventricular depolarization proceeds from endocardium to epicardium.

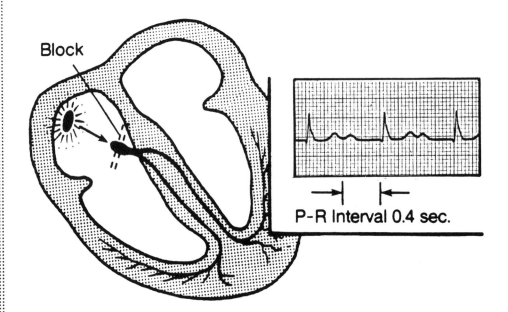

Atrioventricular Conduction Disturbances

First Degree A-V Block

Block

P-R Interval 0.4 sec.

Prolongation of P-R Interval >0.2 sec.

First degree atrioventricular (1° A-V) block represents a delay in the transmission of impulses from the atria to the ventricles. The delay commonly occurs in the A-V node but may occur below it. *A prolonged P-R interval (greater than 0.2 sec.)* is seen on this electrocardiogram.

First degree A-V block represents a delay in the transmission of impulses from the _____ to the _____ .	atria ventricles
The delay in 1° A-V block commonly occurs in the _____ _____ .	A-V node

Second Degree A-V Block

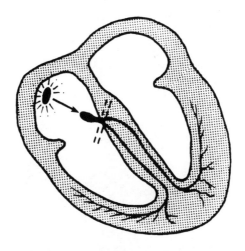

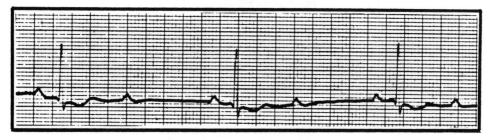

2:1 A-V Block

When the ventricles do not respond to atrial stimuli, the P wave is not followed by a QRS complex. The various grades of *second degree atrioventricular (2° A-V) block* are recognized by the frequency and characteristics of blocked atrial conduction. Seen above are two atrial deflections for every ventricular deflection, or 2:1 A-V block. The atrial rate is 62 and the ventricular rate is 31 beats per min. Three and four P waves for every QRS complex would be known as 3:1 and 4:1 A-V block, respectively. Other examples of 2° A-V block including Mobitz I and II blocks are studied on the following pages.

In second degree A-V block:

some P waves are not followed by ＿＿＿ ＿＿＿＿ .   QRS complexes

when only every second P wave is followed by a QRS complex
we have ＿＿ ＿＿ ＿＿＿ .   2:1 A-V block

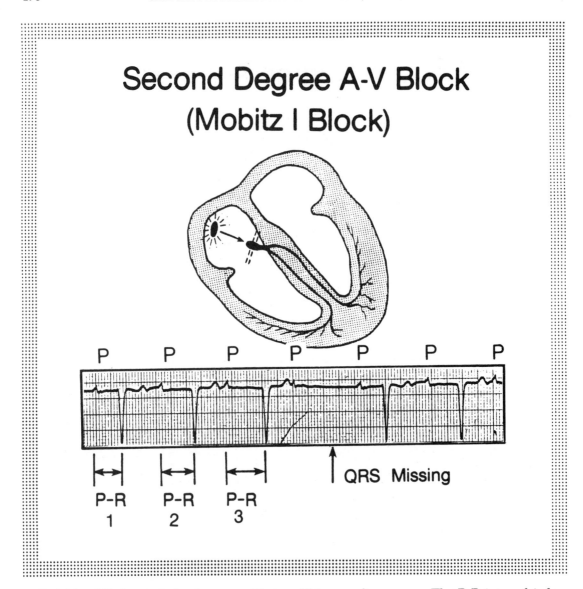

Second Degree A-V Block
(Mobitz I Block)

P   P   P   P   P   P   P

QRS Missing

P-R   P-R   P-R
 1   2   3

In Mobitz I block ventricular beats are "dropped" in a cyclic manner. The P-R interval is less prolonged at first but becomes progressively longer, until an atrial contraction no longer initiates a ventricular response. The cycle is then resumed. In the above electrocardiogram, the first P-R interval is shorter than the second, which is shorter than the third. The fourth P wave does not conduct and is therefore not followed by a QRS complex. The fifth P wave starts the cycle again. This is a typical "Wenckebach" period with progressive lengthening of conduction time ending in a dropped beat. The site of block is usually the A-V node.

In a Wenckebach period there is progressive _____ of   **lengthening**
A-V conduction time ending in a "dropped" beat.

The site of block in Mobitz type I A-V block is usually
the _____ _____ .   **A-V node**

> The ladder diagram of Mobitz type I A-V block (in addition to other leads from the same patient) is illlsutrated on page 371.

Second Degree A-V Block
(Mobitz II Block)

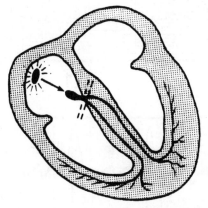

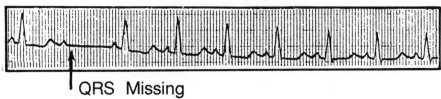

↑ QRS Missing

1. QRS Complex Suddenly Missing
2. P-R Intervals Unchanged

Mobitz type II A-V block is classified under second degree A-V block because P waves are periodically not followed by QRS complexes (arrow). Electrophysiologic studies have shown that the site of block is below the A-V node and is a warning of future complete A-V block. The P-R intervals in the consecutively conducted beats are unchanged, and P waves are periodically and unexpectedly not followed by QRS complexes.

In Mobitz type A-V block:
　the P-R intervals in the consecutively conducted beats
　are _____ , and P waves are periodically and　　　　　**unchanged**
　unexpectedly _____ _____ by QRS complexes.　　**not followed**

　the site of block is below the ____ _____ .　　　　　　　　**A-V node**

> The ladder diagram of Mobitz type II A-V block in this patient is illustrated on page 372.

> The Wenckebach period in *S-A block* is illustrated on page 373.

Second Degree A-V Block

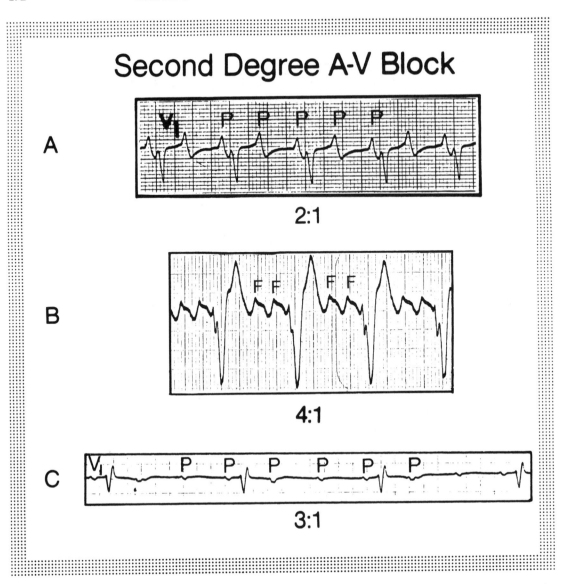

A

2:1

B

4:1

C

3:1

Above are two, three, and four atrial deflections (P waves or flutter waves) for every ventricular deflection (QRS complex). Conduction ratios, e.g., 2:1, 3:1, and 4:1, should not be emphasized at the expense of *rate*. A conduction ratio of 2:1, as in the example on page 169, with an atrial rate of 62 and a dangerously low ventricular rate of 31, is in sharp contrast with (A) and (B) above. Here atrial rates of 150 and 300 result in ventricular rates of 75 with conduction ratios of 2:1 and 4:1. In these two cases (A and B), the A-V node is actually protecting the heart by not allowing every impulse to be transmitted to the ventricles; the heart is protected by the conduction ratio. In C, which is an example of high grade, or advanced, A-V block, the heart is compromised by a low ventricular rate with a conduction ratio frequently 3:1 or greater.

In high grade or advanced A-V block:
   the ventricular rate is usually _____ .   **low**

   the conduction ratio is frequently _____ or greater.   **3:1**

Third Degree (Complete) A-V Block

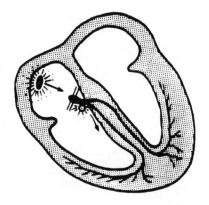

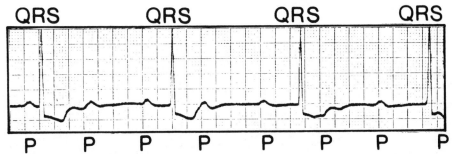

QRS   QRS   QRS   QRS

P   P   P   P   P   P   P   P

Atrial Rate (S-A Node) = 75
Ventricular Rate (A-V Junction) = 33

In *third degree,* or *complete A-V block,* there is no relationship between the atria and the ventricles. The atria, remaining under the control of the S-A node, are beating at 75 per min. and are completely dissociated from the ventricles. Depending on the site of impulse formation, the QRS complexes may be of normal duration, as above, with the pacemaker in the A-V junction, or quite wide and bizarre, with the pacemaker low in the ventricles. The ventricular rate is 33 per min.

In third degree (complete) A-V block:
   there is no relationship between the _____ _____ and the QRS   P waves
   complexes.

   the ventricular rhythm is generally _____ .   regular

> The differences between A-V block and A-V dissociation are presented on page 374.

Pacemaker Therapy

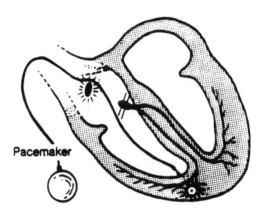

Pacemaker

Pacemaker Impulses

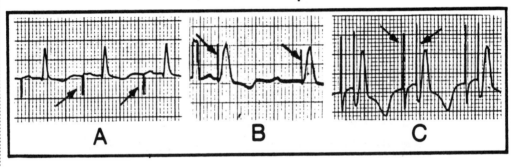

A   B   C

Artificial pacemaker therapy has improved the lives of many patients whose intrinsic systems have faltered or failed completely. A patient with complete A-V block may present with systems of cerebral insufficiency, such as dizziness or clouded mentation, or may actually have lost consciousness because of the low heart rate and poor cardiac output or transient ventricular standstill or fibrillation (Adams-Stokes syndrome). The present day treatment is pacemaker therapy to maintain a proper heart rate and good cardiac output. The arrows point to pacemaker impulses.

    A. Atrial pacing with a pacemaker impulse stimulating atrial depolarization.

    B. Ventricular pacing with a pacemaker impulse stimulating ventricular depolarization.

    C. Atrial and ventricular pacing with pacemaker impulses stimulating both atria and ventricles at set intervals.

Pacemaker therapy is introduced here to illustrate various electrocardiographic manifestations of the pacemaker impulse. For complete understanding of this remarkable achievement in medical therapy please consult the references.[17-20]

A patient who develops high grade or complete A-V block requires _____ therapy.   pacemaker

The sudden loss of consciousness as a result of ventricular standstill or fibrillation is known as the _____ syndrome.   Adams-Stokes

Intraventricular Conduction Disturbances

Bundle Branch Block

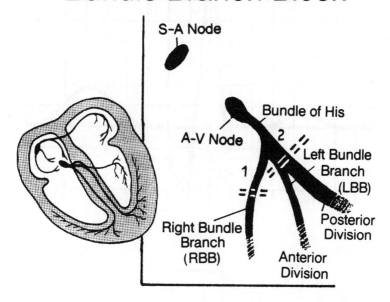

1. Right Bundle Branch Block (RBBB)

2. Left Bundle Branch Block (LBBB)

Bundle branch block refers to an interference with conduction in either the right bundle branch or the left bundle branch. The left bundle branch is very short and branches early into an anterior and a posterior division. The right bundle branch, on the other hand, continues almost to the apex of the right ventricle before branching.

Bundle branch block refers to a block in either _____ or _____ bundle branches.   right
                                                                                                  left

The left bundle branch divides early into _____ and _____ divisions.   anterior
                                                                                            posterior

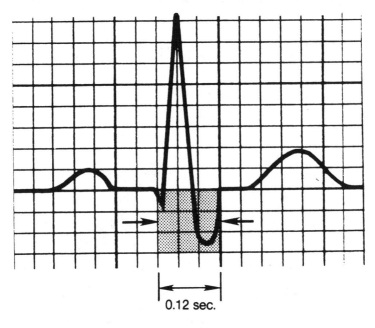

Right Bundle Branch Block

0.12 sec.

1. QRS Interval 0.12 sec. or Greater

The conduction system is similar to a series of superhighways over which the electrical impulse travels. If there is a block in any of these pathways, as above, in *right bundle branch block (RBBB)*, the impulse has to travel through tissue outside the normal pathways of conduction, with delay in conduction. A delay in depolarization therefore results in a *prolongation of the QRS interval* (QRS complex duration). In RBBB, the delay affects only the terminal portion of the QRS complex.

In RBBB there is prolongation of the _____ _____ .   QRS complex

Only the _____ portion of the QRS complex is   terminal
affected by RBBB.

Right Bundle Branch Block

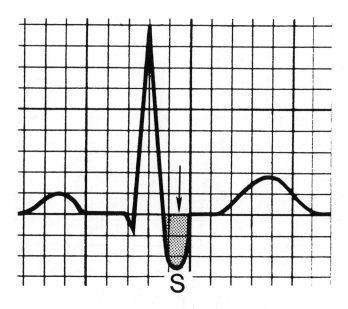

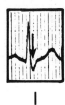

I

2. S Wave Present in Lead I

Regardless of where the block may be in right bundle branch block, early depolarization will already have occurred. Only the *terminal* QRS vector is affected by right bundle branch block (RBBB), as mentioned on page 176. This is important, since the electrocardiographic manifestations of initial QRS vector abnormalities, such as the Q waves in myocardial infarction, are not obscured. This *terminal delay* is to the *right,* inscribing the S wave in lead I.

The initial QRS vector is _____ affected by RBBB.   **not**

The terminal QRS vector delay inscribes a(n) ____ wave in lead I.   **S**

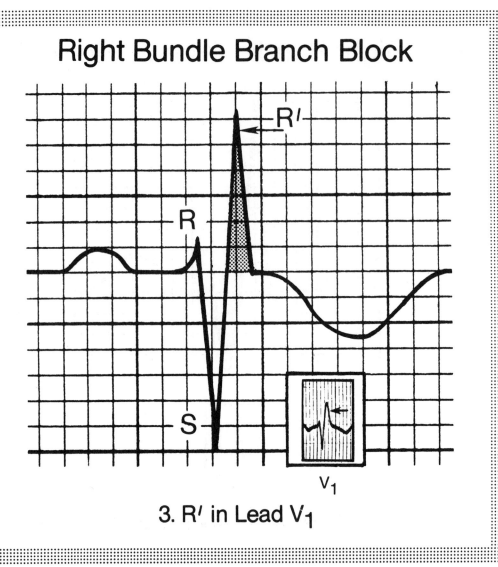

Right Bundle Branch Block

3. R′ in Lead V₁

The *terminal* QRS vector, which is affected by right bundle branch block (RBBB), is not only to the right, resulting in an *S wave in lead I*, but also *anterior*, producing a second R wave known as an *R′ in lead V₁*. The terminal QRS vector moves toward lead V_1.

Because the initial portion of the QRS vector is not affected by RBBB,
the _____ _____ of myocardial infarction are not obscured.   Q waves

The terminal anterior QRS vector inscribes a terminal R wave
or _____ wave on the electrocardiogram.   R′

Right Bundle Branch Block

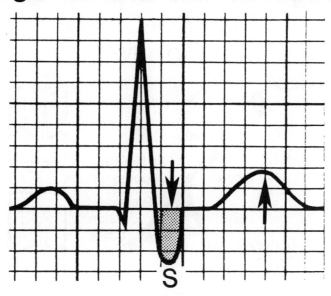

S

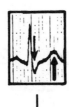

I

4. Repolarization Abnormalities

Right bundle branch block (RBBB) is accompanied by repolarization abnormalities. These are *secondary* to abnormal depolarization. The T wave orientation is opposite in direction to the *terminal* deflection of the QRS complex. Thus, in lead I, with a terminal S wave, the T wave is upright, and in lead V_1, with a terminal R or R' wave, the T wave is negative. If this relationship is not found, then primary repolarization abnormalities are evident in addition to the RBBB.

In RBBB:

repolarization abnormalities are usually _____ to   secondary
abnormal depolarization.

the T wave orientation is usually opposite in direction to
the _____ deflection of the QRS complex.   terminal

Right Bundle Branch Block
Principal Criteria
Review

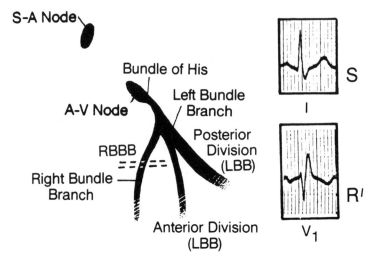

1. QRS Interval 0.12 sec. or Greater
2. S Wave in Lead I
3. R′ in Lead V₁
4. Repolarization Abnormalities

Review

Right bundle branch block (RBBB) is easily recognized by these four characteristics. RBBB may be found as a congenital condition without any clinical evidence of heart disease. It may also be found in association with an enlarged right ventricle, myocardial infarction, and hypertensive cardiovascular disease.

In summary, the principal findings in RBBB are:

1. _____   QRS interval 0.12 sec. or more
2. _____   S wave in lead I
3. _____   R′ in lead V₁
4. _____   Repolarization abnormalities

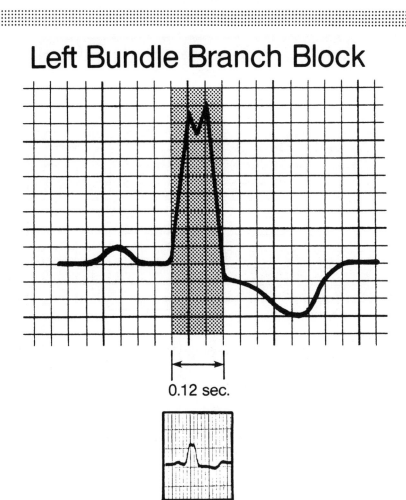

Left Bundle Branch Block

0.12 sec.

1. QRS Interval 0.12 sec. or Greater

In *left bundle branch block (LBBB)*, as in right bundle branch block, the QRS complex is prolonged. The delay in conduction is caused by the block, with the electrical impulse having been forced to travel outside the normal pathways of conduction where conduction is slower. In LBBB, both the initial and terminal QRS vectors are affected.

In LBBB:
as in RBBB, there is prolongation of the _____ _____ .   QRS complex

both the _____ and _____ QRS vectors   initial terminal
are affected.

Left Bundle Branch Block

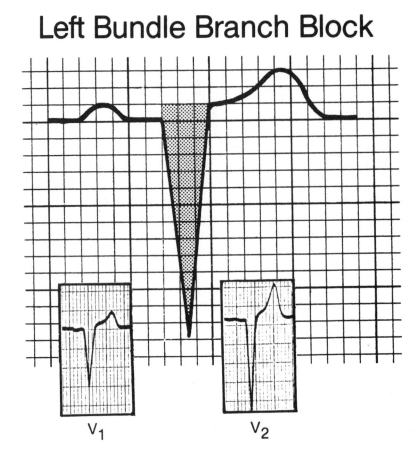

V_1 V_2

2a. QRS Complex Predominantly or Entirely Negative in Leads V_1 and V_2.

In left bundle branch block (LBBB), in contrast with right bundle branch block, the entire sequence of ventricular depolarization is altered. Both the initial and terminal QRS vectorial forces point more *leftward* and *posteriorly* in comparison with the findings in normal conduction. Therefore, the initial *R waves* seen in the normal electrocardiogram in leads V_1, V_2, and V_3 are much smaller and have often disappeared in leads V_1 and V_2, simulating anterior myocardial infarction. Left ventricular hypertrophy may also be simulated because of the size of the complexes.

In LBBB:
the normal initial R waves in leads _____ , V_1
_____ , and _____ are much smaller or have V_2 V_3
disappeared.
the disappearance of the initial R waves in the
right precordial leads
simulates _____ _____   **anterior myocardial**

_____ .   **infarction**

Left Bundle Branch Block

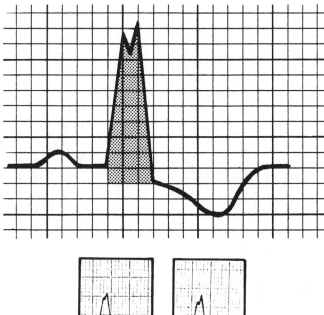

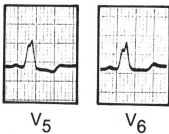

V₅ V₆

2b. QRS Complex Predominantly Positive in Leads V5 and V6 and Often Notched

The mean QRS vector, oriented more leftward and posteriorly, which causes leads V_1 and V_2 to be predominantly or entirely *negative,* causes leads V_5 and V_6 to be predominantly or entirely *positive.* The QRS complex in these leads is often notched. Left bundle branch block (LBBB) is often associated with organic disease of the left ventricle.

In LBBB:

the more leftward and posterior vector causes leads V_5 and V_6 to be predominantly or entirely _____ .

positive

does not often occur in the _____ heart.

normal

Left Bundle Branch Block

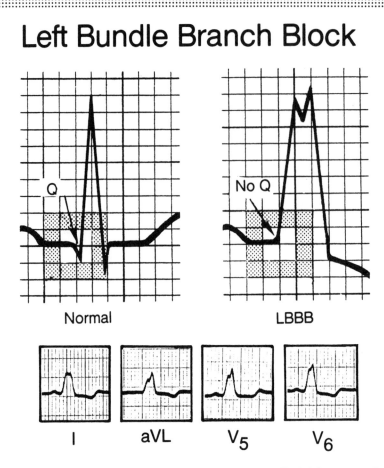

Normal   LBBB

I   aVL   V5   V6

3. Absence of Small, Normal, Q Waves in Leads I , aVL, V5 and V6.

With the more leftward orientation of the mean QRS vector, the *small* Q waves *normally* seen in leads I, aVL, V_5, and V_6 disappear. The Q waves of a well-documented myocardial infarction may disappear with the onset of left bundle branch block (LBBB), masking the electrocardiographic evidence of the infarction. Nevertheless, acute myocardial infarction may be recognized even in the presence of LBBB. See pages 308 and 309.

In LBBB

the small _____ _____ , normally seen in leads I, aVL, V_5, and V_6,   **Q waves**
disappear.

the Q waves of myocardial infarction may be _____ .   **masked**

> Myocardial infarction in the presence of LBBB is presented on pages 308 and 309.

Left Bundle Branch Block

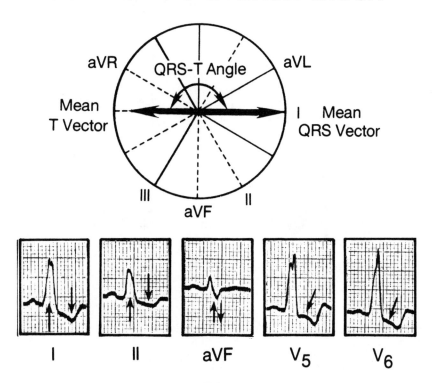

4. Repolarization Abnormalities
a. S-T Segment Depression
b. Wide QRS-T Angle

The repolarization alterations occurring with left bundle branch block (LBBB) may be marked. Note that where the QRS complex is positive the T wave is negative, and the transition is shared at lead aVF. The QRS-T angle, is therefore, very wide and the S-T segment is depressed.

In LBBB, the repolarization abnormalities
electrocardiographically inscribe the following:

1. _____

2. _____

S-T segment depression
Wide QRS-T angle

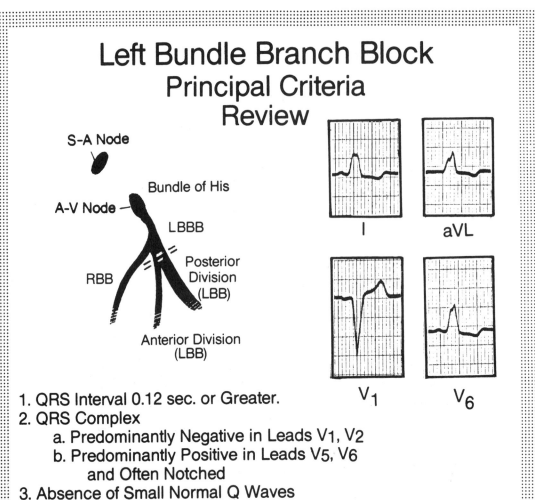

Left Bundle Branch Block
Principal Criteria
Review

1. QRS Interval 0.12 sec. or Greater.
2. QRS Complex
   a. Predominantly Negative in Leads V1, V2
   b. Predominantly Positive in Leads V5, V6
      and Often Notched
3. Absence of Small Normal Q Waves
      in Leads I, aVL, V5 and V6
4. Repolarization Abnormalities

Review

Do not make the diagnosis of anterior or anteroseptal myocardial infarction from the lack of R waves in the right precordial leads in the presence of left bundle branch block (LBBB). In addition, do not exclude the diagnosis of myocardial infarction in the presence of LBBB. Owing to the size of the complexes, especially leads V_1 and V_2, left ventricular hypertrophy may be simulated by LBBB.

In summary, the principal electrocardiographic findings in LBBB include:

1. _____   QRS interval 0.12 sec. or greater
2. _____   QRS complex:
                                Predominantly negative in leads V_1 and V_2
                                Predominantly positive in leads V_5 and V_6
                                and often notched
3. _____   Absence of small normal Q waves in leads I,
                                aVL, V_5, and V_6
4. _____   Repolarization abnormalities

The Hemiblocks

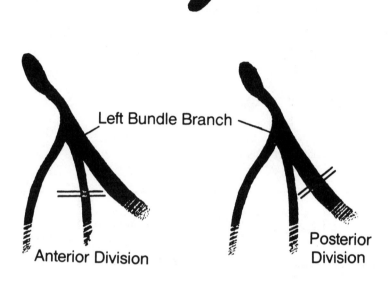

Left Bundle Branch

Anterior Division

Posterior Division

Left Anterior Hemiblock (LAH)

Left Posterior Hemiblock (LPH)

As noted earlier, the left bundle branch is short and branches early into an anterior and a posterior division. The term *hemiblock* refers to a block in either of the two divisions, the anterior *(left anterior hemiblock, LAH)* or the posterior *(left posterior hemiblock, LPH)*.

Hemiblock refers to a block in either the _____
or _____**division of the left bundle branch.**

anterior
posterior

The two types of hemiblock are:
   1. _____
   2. _____

LAH
LPH

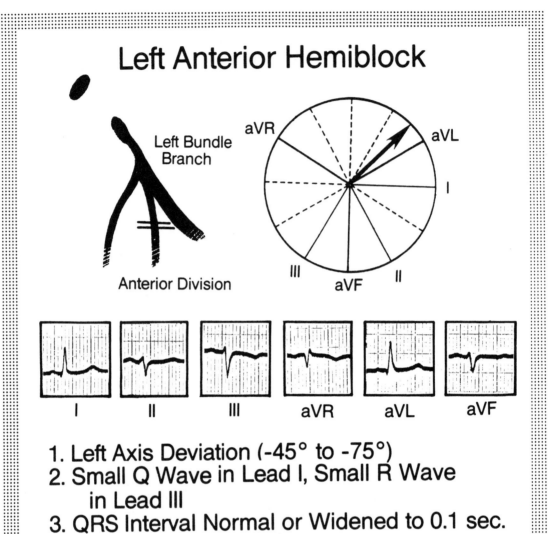

Left Anterior Hemiblock

Left Bundle Branch

Anterior Division

aVR   aVL   I   III   aVF   II

I   II   III   aVR   aVL   aVF

1. Left Axis Deviation (-45° to -75°)
2. Small Q Wave in Lead I, Small R Wave in Lead III
3. QRS Interval Normal or Widened to 0.1 sec.

Left anterior hemiblock, a conduction disturbance in the anterior division of the left bundle branch, is characterized by a marked *left axis deviation* of the mean QRS vector. Note that the QRS complexes in leads II and aVF are predominantly negative, with lead I positive. The QRS complex may be normal or only minimally widened, since a pathway of conduction still remains intact for the electrical impulse to traverse without passage through myocardial tissue.

The findings in left anterior hemiblock include:

1. _____
2. _____
3. _____

Left axis deviation
Small Q_I, small R_{III}
QRS interval 0.1 sec. or less

Left Posterior Hemiblock

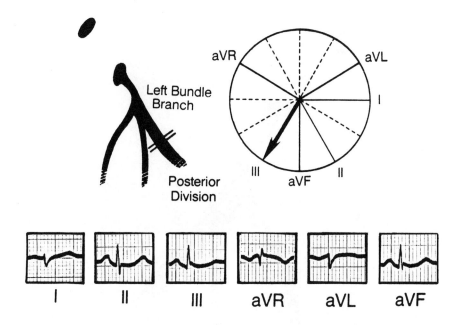

Left Bundle Branch

Posterior Division

aVR aVL I III aVF II

| I | II | III | aVR | aVL | aVF |

1. Right Axis Deviation
2. Small R Wave in Lead I, Small Q Wave in Lead III
3. QRS Interval Normal or Widened to 0.1 sec.
4. No Evidence of Right Ventricular Hypertrophy

In *left posterior hemiblock* the mean QRS vector is deviated to the *right*. Note the right axis deviation, with the QRS complex almost entirely negative in lead I. There should be no evidence of right ventricular hypertrophy when making the diagnosis of left posterior hemiblock. Right ventricular hypertrophy may also cause marked right axis deviation.

The findings in left posterior hemiblock include:

1. _____   Right axis deviation
2. _____   Small R wave in lead I, small Q wave in lead III
3. _____   QRS interval normal or widened to 0.1 sec.
4. _____   No evidence of right ventricular hypertrophy

The Trifascicular System

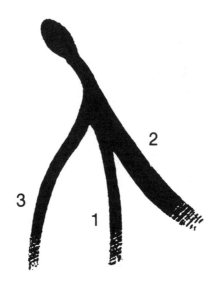

1. Anterior Division of Left Bundle Branch
2. Posterior Division of Left Bundle Branch
3. Right Bundle Branch

Both divisions of the left bundle branch plus the right bundle branch constitute the *trifascicular* system of intraventricular conduction. Each of the three component parts is called a fascicle. Block in two of the three fascicles is commonly seen and is known as bifascicular block.

The trifascicular system is composed of:

1. _____   Anterior division, left bundle branch
2. _____   Posterior division, left bundle branch
3. _____   Right bundle branch

Bifascicular Block Types

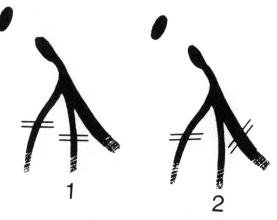

1

2

1. Right Bundle Branch Block plus Left Anterior Hemiblock
RBBB + LAH

2. Right Bundle Branch Block plus Left Posterior Hemiblock
RBBB + LPH

Right bundle branch block plus left anterior hemiblock (RBBB + LAH) or right bundle branch block plus left posterior hemiblock (RBBB + LPH) each involves two of the three fascicles and has been termed *bifascicular* block. Block in all three fascicles would result in complete atrioventricular block.

Block in two of the three fascicles is known as _____**block.**   bifascicular

Two types of bifascicular block are:

   1. _____   **RBBB + LAH**
   2. _____   **RBBB + LPH**

Bifascicular Block
RBBB + LAH

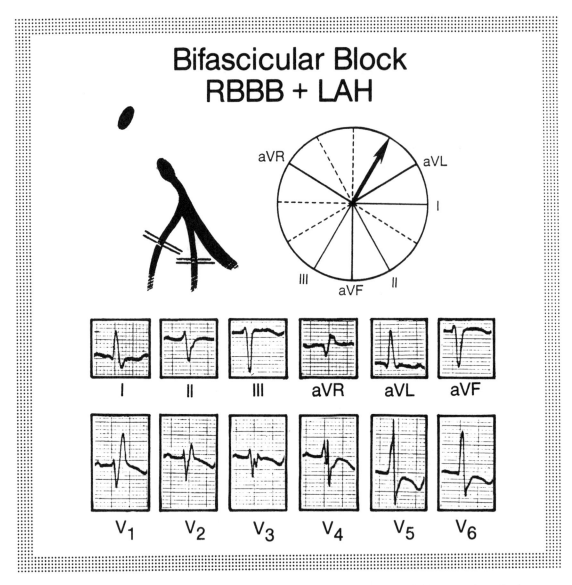

The combination of *right bundle branch block plus left anterior hemiblock (RBBB + LAH, also known as left anterior fascicular block)* is frequently seen. This condition often does not progress to complete atrioventricular block, since the posterior division is a sturdy branch with a dual blood supply. Note the typical right bundle branch block associated with left axis deviation.

The posterior fascicle of the left bundle branch has a(n) _____   dual
blood supply.

Therefore, RBBB + LAH does not usually progress to _____   complete
A-V block.

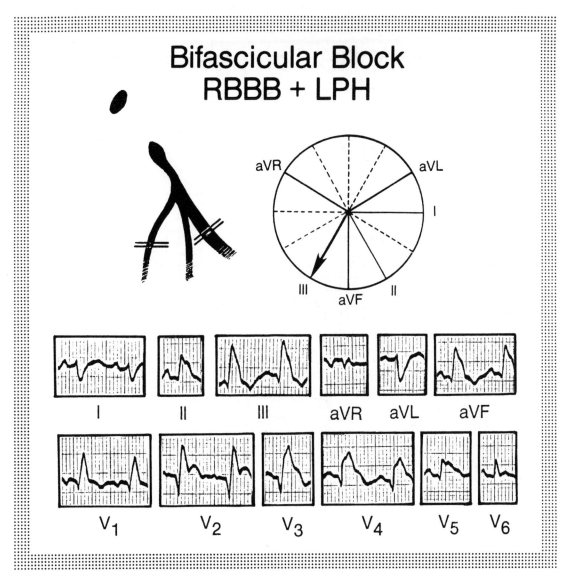

Bifascicular Block
RBBB + LPH

The combination of *right bundle branch block plus left posterior hemiblock (RBBB + LPH, left posterior fascicular block)* may augur ill for the patient, since in this disorder the entire atrioventricular conduction system is dependent on the weakest fascicle, the anterior division, with a single blood supply. These patients must be followed closely; pacemaker therapy must be considered with progress of the disease to the third fascicle. This patient also had an anterior myocardial infarction; hence the initial Q waves in the precordial leads.

The anterior fascicle of the left bundle branch is a thin fascicle with
a _____ blood supply.   single

Therefore, in RBBB + _____, the entire A-V conduction system may   LPH
be in jeopardy.

Wide QRS Complexes With Supraventricular Pacemaker
Wolff-Parkinson-White (W-P-W) Syndrome

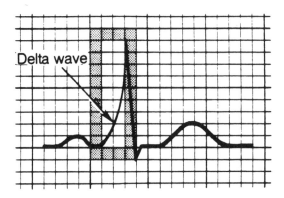

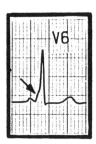

Another example of a wide QRS complex with a supraventricular pacemaker is the *Wolff-Parkinson-White (W-P-W) syndrome.* The W-P-W syndrome represents an anomalous pathway or bypass from the atria to the ventricles. Because patients with the syndrome may be subject to attacks of paroxysmal tachycardia, it is included in the study of arrhythmias. The electrocardiographic characteristics, which may be present only intermittently, include:

1. Short P-R interval (0.12 sec. or less).
2. Prolonged QRS interval (greater than 0.1 sec.).
3. Slurring of the upstroke by a *delta* wave.

In the W-P-W syndrome the slurred initial component of the QRS complex is known as the _____ wave.	delta
The delta wave may be present only _____ .	intermittently

> An example of rate dependent LBBB, which may be mistaken for the W-P-W syndrome, is illustrated on page 375.

L-G-L Syndrome

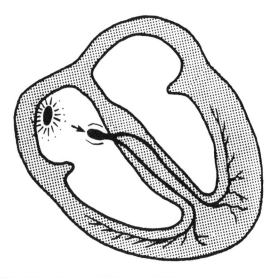

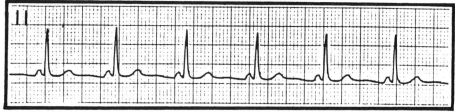

The syndrome of the short P-R interval with the normal QRS complex was described by Loun, Ganong, and Levine (L-G-L syndrome). Paroxysmal rapid heart action has been associated with this syndrome. Both the W-P-W and L-G-L syndromes are classified under the heading of "pre-excitation."

The W-P-W and L-G-L syndromes:
   have been associated with episodes of _____ .   **tachycardia**

   are classified under the heading of _____ .   **pre-excitation**

> The pre-excitation syndromes (W-P-W and L-G-L) are further discussed on pages 394 to 396, including references.

Practice
ECG Analysis

Practice
ECG Analysis

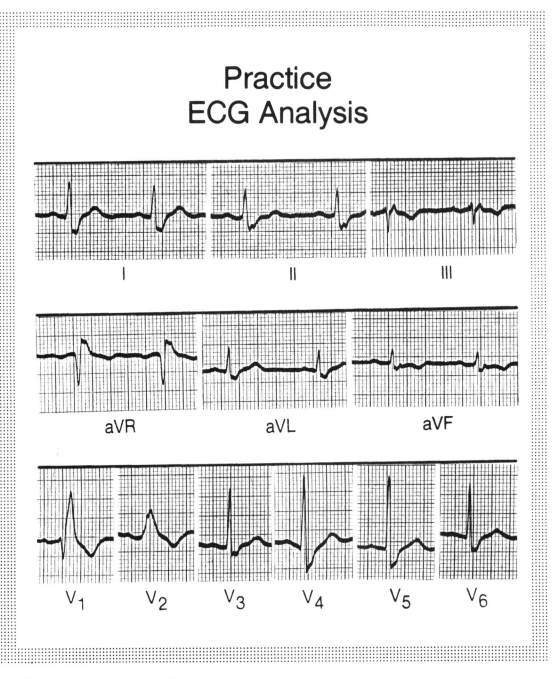

The patient is a 58-year-old asymptomatic man.

Analysis:

ECG ANALYSIS

1. Rhythm and rate
   Rhythm: sinus
   Rate: 65/min.
   P-R Interval: 0.18 sec.
2. QRS complex
   Duration: 0.18 sec.
   Axis: $+15°$
   QRS complex wide, with an S wave in lead I and an R′ in lead V_1
3. Ventricular repolarization
   S-T segment: neither significantly elevated nor depressed
   T wave: opposite in direction to the terminal deflection of the QRS complex seen best in leads I, II, III, V_1, V_4 to V_6
4. Q-T interval:
   0.42 sec.

Impression and Comments

Sinus rhythm
Right bundle branch block (RBBB)
Ventricular repolarization abnormalities (secondary to RBBB)
   Note the RBBB criteria:
   1. The wide QRS interval
   2. S wave in lead I
   3. R′ in lead V_1
   4. Ventricular repolarization abnormalities

Practice
ECG Analysis

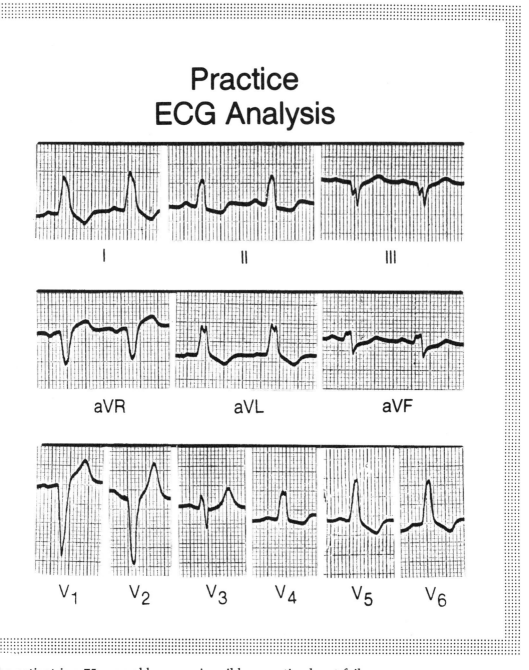

The patient is a 75-year-old woman in mild congestive heart failure.

Analysis:

ECG ANALYSIS

1. Rhythm and rate
   Rhythm: sinus
   Rate: 83/min.
   P-R Interval: 0.18 sec.
2. QRS complex
   Duration: 0.14 sec.
   Axis: 0°
   QS complexes in leads V_1 and V_2
   Absence of the small normal Q waves in leads I, aVL, V_5, and V_6
3. Ventricular repolarization
   S-T segment: depressed in leads I, II, aVL, V_5, and V_6
   T wave: inverted in leads I, II, aVL, V_5, and V_6, wide QRS-T angle
4. Q-T interval:
   0.38 sec.

Impression and Comments

Sinus rhythm
Left bundle branch block (LBBB)
Ventricular repolarization abnormalities
   Review the LBBB criteria present here:
   1. The wide QRS interval
   2. QS complexes in leads V_1 and V_2
   3. Absence of the small normal Q waves in leads I, aVL, V_5, and V_6
   4. Ventricular repolarization abnormalities

Chapter 6

Arrhythmias

In previous chapters we studied the 12-lead electrocardiogram using leads I, II, III, aVR, aVL, aVF, and V_1 to V_6. In the monitoring of arrhythmias, single leads are often used, in addition to the 12-lead electrocardiogram. The single leads commonly used are leads II (modified), MCL_1, and MCL_6. Lead II is a modified lead II since the positive and negative electrodes are not placed on the respective extremities, but on the chest. In lead MCL_1 the positive electrode is placed on the chest in the position of lead V_1. In lead MCL_6 the positive electrode is placed on the chest in the position of lead V_6. These leads are illustrated on pages 376 and 377.

> The leads commonly used to monitor arrhythmias are illustrated on pages 376 and 377.

Electrical Conduction System
of the Heart
Review

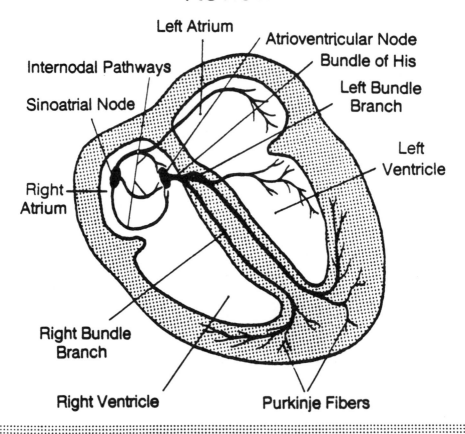

Left Atrium

Atrioventricular Node

Bundle of His

Internodal Pathways

Left Bundle
Branch

Sinoatrial Node

Left
Ventricle

Right
Atrium

Right Bundle
Branch

Right Ventricle

Purkinje Fibers

Review

The electrical conduction system of the heart was first illustrated on page 6. The normal site of impulse formation in the heart is the *sinoatrial (S-A) node.* After the atria are depolarized, the impulse spreads through the *atrioventricular (A-V) node* and *bundle of His* to the *left (LBB) and right (RBB) bundle branches* and then to the ventricular muscle through the *Purkinje network,* leading to ventricular depolarization.

Following depolarization of the atria the impulse spreads to the _____ node, bundle of _____ and bundle _____, then through the _____ network.

A-V His
branches Purkinje

Rate of Impulse Formation
(Impulses Per Minute)
Review

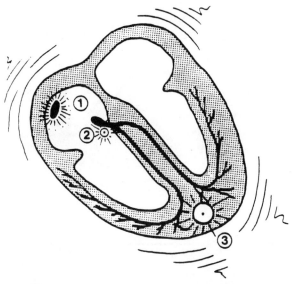

① S-A Node   60-100

② A-V Junction 40-60

③ Ventricle   20-40

Review

Although the primary and dominant pacemaker of the heart is the *S-A node,* under various circumstances and stimuli another pacemaker may become dominant. Each pacemaker has its own inherent rate. The pacemaker with the fastest inherent rate is usually the dominant pacemaker.

The rates of impulse formation (impulses per minute) are as follows:

1. S-A node: _____ to _____   60-100
2. A-V junction: _____ to _____   40-60
3. Ventricle: _____ to _____   20-40

Normal Sinus Rhythm

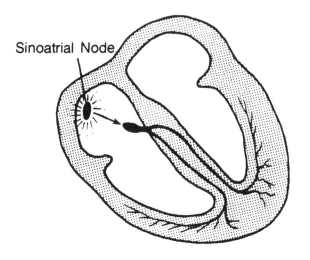

Sinoatrial Node

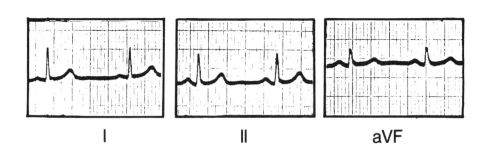

I   II   aVF

Before examining rhythm disturbances, let us review the criteria for *normal sinus rhythm.*

1. The mean P vector is normal (the P waves are constant and upright in leads I, II, and aVF).
2. Each P wave is followed by a QRS complex, and each QRS complex is preceded by a P wave.
3. The P-R interval is from 0.12 to 0.20 sec. (three to five small boxes wide) and constant from beat to beat.
4. The rate is regular, between 60 and 100 beats per min.

When the word "nodal" is used it refers to the *A-V* node and *not* to the S-A node. Any beat or rhythm originating outside the *S-A node* is an *ectopic* beat or rhythm, ectopic in that it does not originate in the normal site.

The heart rate in normal sinus rhythm is _____ to _____   **60 100**
per min.

A rhythm originating outside the S-A node is an _____   **ectopic**
rhythm.

> The ladder diagram or "laddergram" is a useful aid in the study of normal and abnormal rhythms of the heart. Review it on pages 356 and 357.

Sinus Tachycardia

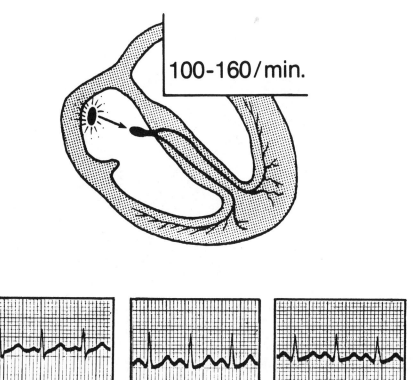

100-160/min.

I   II   aVF

If all the criteria for normal sinus rhythm have been fulfilled but the heart rate is greater than 100 beats per min., the rhythm is called *sinus tachycardia.* Tachycardia means fast heart. The heart rate in sinus tachycardia is 100 to 160 per min. The word sinus appearing before the tachycardia indicates that the origin of the rhythm is the S-A node, the normal pacemaker of the heart.

Tachycardia means _____ _____ .   **fast heart**

In sinus tachycardia the heart rate is _____ to _____   **100 160**
per min. and the origin of the impulse is the _____ _____ .   **S-A node**

Sinus Bradycardia

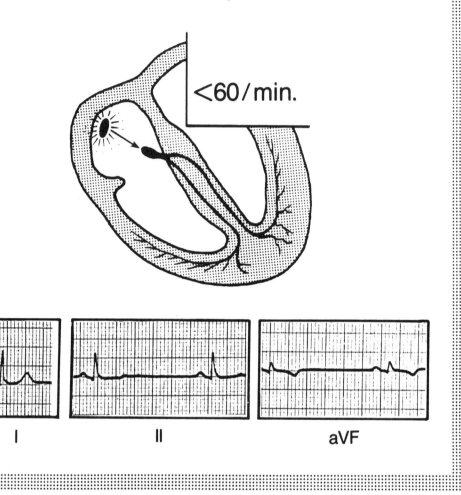

I   II   aVF

If the heart rate is under 60 beats per min. but all the criteria for normal sinus rhythm have been fulfilled, the rhythm is known as *sinus bradycardia*. Bradycardia means slow heart.

Bradycardia means _____ _____ .	**slow heart**
In sinus bradycardia the heart rate is less than _____ per min.	**60**
and the P waves are positive and uniform in lead _____ .	**II**

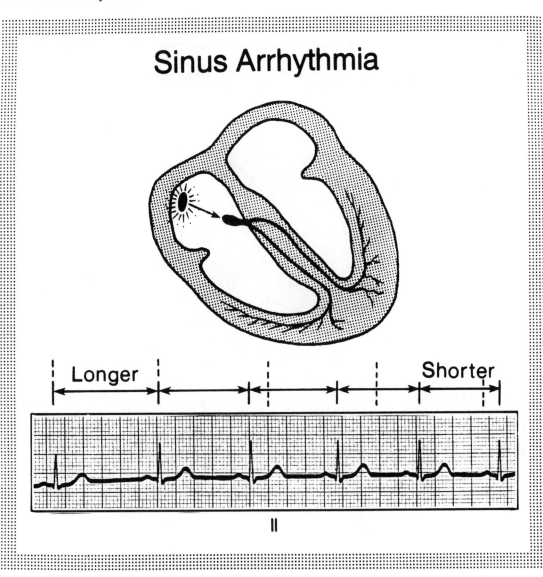

Sinus Arrhythmia

Longer

Shorter

II

Sinus arrhythmia meets all the criteria described under normal sinus rhythm except for the variation in rate, often associated with the respiratory cycles. It is commonly seen in young people. The P-R intervals are constant, but the R-R intervals are continually changing. The heart rate in this electrocardiogram varies from 53 to 68 beats per min., more than 10%.

Sinus arrhythmia is common in _____ _____ .   **young people**

Although the _____ intervals are stable,   **P-R**
the _____ intervals are constantly changing.   **R-R**

> Complete the ladder diagram of sinus arrhythmia on page 378.

Sinoatrial (S-A) Block

II

In *sinoatrial (S-A) block,* the S-A node initiates the impulse but the *propagation* is blocked, so that the atria are not depolarized and, therefore, there is no P wave. S-A block represents a failure of impulse propagation rather than of impulse formation. The pause is a multiple of the regular cycle length. The block, represented by the letter B above (arrow), is seen where the P should normally be. *Block* refers to a delay or interruption of conduction of an impulse.

_____ refers to a delay or interruption of the conduction   **Block**
of an impulse.

In S-A block the _____ _____ initiates an impulse but   **S-A node**
the _____ of the impulse, however, is blocked, and   **propagation**
the pause is a _____ of the regular P-P interval.   **multiple**

> The ladder diagram of S-A block (in addition to other electrocardiographic tracings from the same patient) is
  illustrated on page 379.

Sinus Arrest

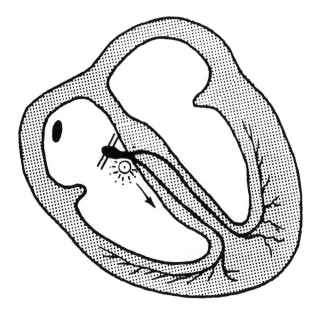

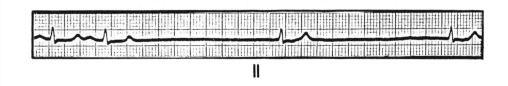

II

Sinus arrest is a sudden failure of the S-A node to initiate an expected impulse, which is one manifestation of the "sick sinus" syndrome. Often the long pauses follow periods of rapid heart rate. Fortunately, a lower pacemaker often becomes dominant, initiating a new rhythm. The new rhythm, following the sinus arrest, is known as an *escape* rhythm (in this case A-V junctional, to be described shortly).

In sinus arrest the _____ _____ fails to initiate an impulse.   S-A node

The new rhythm is known as a(n) _____ rhythm.   escape

Premature Atrial Contraction (PAC)

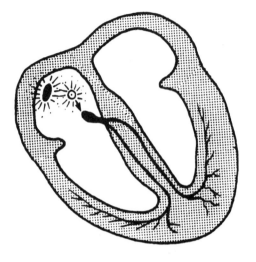

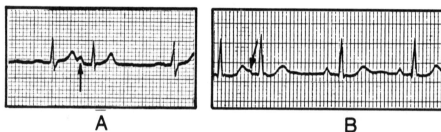

A   B

Premature contractions (PACs) of the atria are seen when an *ectopic atrial pacemaker* propagates an impulse before the next normal beat is due. The PACs may be conducted to the ventricles, as seen above. The P wave of the PAC differs from the sinus P wave in contour. In general, following PACs, the P-R interval may be normal or prolonged, and the QRS complex may be of normal contour and duration or of changed configuration and prolonged, depending on the state of refractoriness of the conduction tissue. Also, the PACs may herald paroxysms of atrial tachycardia. Note that the P waves (arrows) of the PACs in (A) and (B) are partially hidden within the preceding T waves. The earlier P waves in (B) are more completely hidden.

A PAC originates in a(n) _____ atrial pacemaker, and the P   ectopic
wave of the PAC _____ from the sinus P wave in contour.   differs

PACs may herald paroxysms   atrial
of _____ _____ .   tachycardia

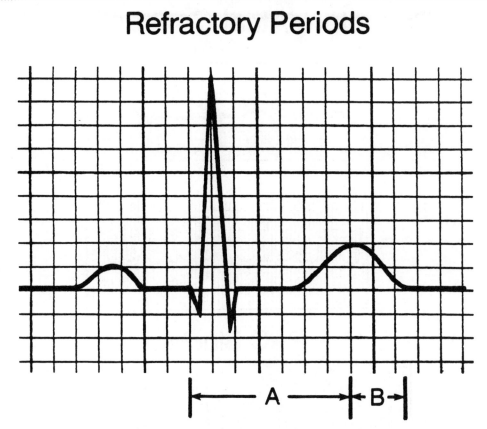

Refractory Periods

A. Absolute Refractory Period
B. Relative Refractory Period

To understand why a PAC is blocked (not conducted), it is important to know when the absolute and relative refractory periods of the ventricle occur. Earlier (pages 4 and 5), the processes of depolarization and repolarization were described. The process of depolarization reflects the flow of an electrical current to all cells along the pathway of conduction. The cells then return to their original resting state by the process of repolarization. Ventricular repolarization is complete at the end of the T wave (pages 13 and 14), permitting a new impulse to start the process again.

A new impulse, occurring before the peak of the T wave, finds the ventricular conduction system unable to accept it. This is the *absolute refractory period.* Although the downslope of the T

Ventricular repolarization is complete at the end of the _____ wave.   T

The period after an impulse when the conduction system cannot be stimulated is the _____ refractory period.   absolute

Premature Atrial Contractions

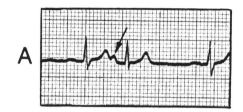

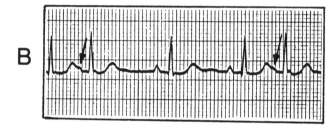

PAC Blocked

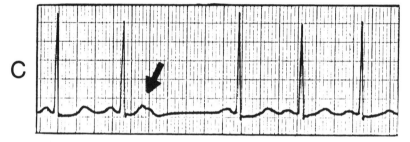

wave is still within the refractory period, an impulse may be conducted under certain circumstances. This is the *relative refractory period*. Note that the PACs in (A) and (B) occur during the relative refractory period and are followed by QRS complexes. In (C), the PAC occurs during the absolute refractory period and is not followed by ventricular depolarization (QRS complex). The PAC is blocked, not conducted.

A PAC that is not followed by a ventricular depolarization (QRS complex) is a _____ PAC.

blocked

Before ventricular depolarization is complete, the period when an impulse, under certain circumstances, may be conducted is the _____ refractory period.

relative

Atrial Tachycardia

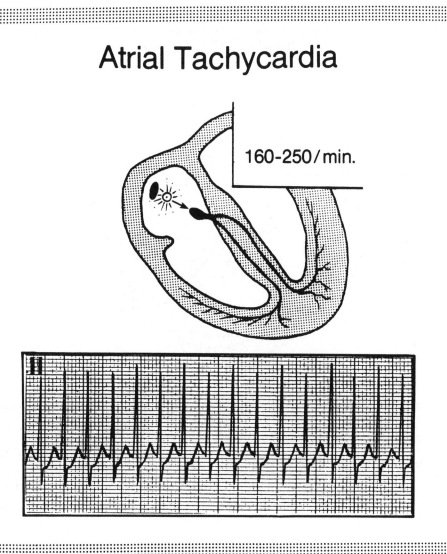

160–250/min.

The S-A node can emit impulses up to approximately 160 per min. in the resting state. If the rate is above 160, another pacemaker must be considered. Here the S-A node is no longer the dominant pacemaker at a rate of 240 per min. *Atrial tachycardia* is characterized by a rapid (160 to 250 per min.) rate and regular rhythm, sudden in onset, often terminating abruptly; it may be followed by a pause. The P waves, when seen, differ from the sinus P waves in contour because the atrial pacemaker is an ectopic pacemaker.

Atrial tachycardia is characterized by an atrial rate of _____ to _____ per min.

160
250

The atrial pacemaker in atrial tachycardia is an _____ pacemaker.

ectopic

> It is important to understand the concept of *reentry* in the study of arrhythmias because it is the mechanism of most supraventricular and many ventricular tachycardias. See pages 380 to 382 for information on *reentry* and *enhanced automaticity*. Review the pre-excitation syndromes, W-P-W and L-G-L, pages 194 and 195, and study pages 382 and 394 to 396.

Atrial Flutter

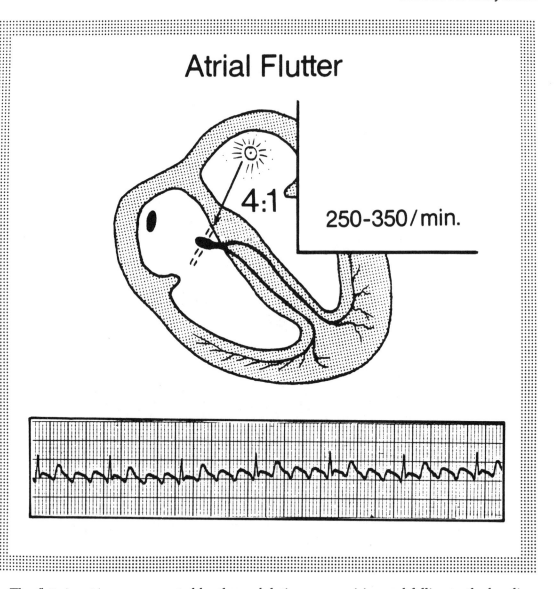

4:1

250-350/min.

The *fluttering atria* are represented by the undulating waves, rising and falling to the baseline. Note the saw-tooth character of the atrial waves (F or flutter waves). The atrial rate is 300 per min., whereas the ventricular rate is 75 per min., with a ratio of 4:1. The atrial rate in atrial flutter is usually 250 to 350 per min. The A-V node protects the ventricles by not allowing every impulse that reaches it to be transmitted to the ventricles (as noted on page 172). Only one of four impulses is reaching the ventricles, as illustrated; hence there is 4:1 A-V conduction.

The atrial rate in atrial flutter is _____ to _____ per min., and the atrial waves often have a _____ appearance.

250 350
saw-tooth

The A-V conduction ratio in this electrocardiogram is _____ .

4:1

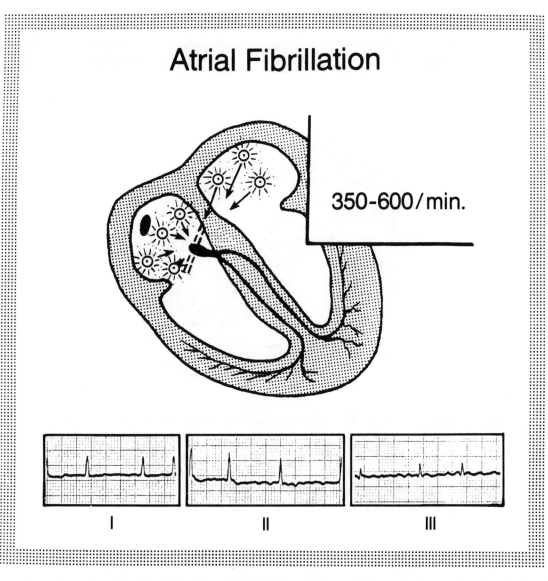

Atrial Fibrillation

350-600/min.

I II III

Disorganized, ineffective contractions of the atria (350 to 600 beats per min.) characterize *atrial fibrillation*. No P waves are seen, and the ventricular response is irregular, depending on how many of the 350 to 600 impulses are conducted to the ventricles. If the atrial rate is 500 per min. and the ventricular rate is 125 per min., it means that one in four atrial impulses is conducted, irregularly, to the ventricles. This rhythm has been described as irregularly irregular.

In atrial fibrillation:
the rhythm is _____ irregular and
no _____ waves are seen.

the atrial rate is _____ to _____ per min.

irregularly
P

350 600

Multifocal Atrial Tachycardia

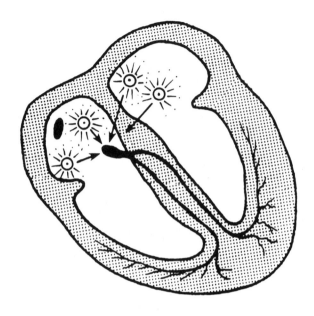

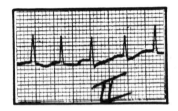

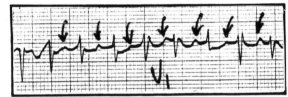

Multifocal (chaotic) atrial tachycardia is sometimes mistaken for atrial fibrillation because the rhythm is also irregularly irregular. At a quick glance, lead II might appear to be an example of atrial fibrillation. Lead V_1, analogous to the monitoring lead MCL_1 (see pages 203 and 376 to 377), however, reveals the different P wave contours as well as the varying P-R intervals. This rhythm is frequently found in patients with chronic obstructive pulmonary disease (COPD) associated with hypoxia. Immediate treatment includes oxygen.

Multifocal atrial tachycardia:

    may be mistaken for _____ _____ .   **atrial fibrillation**

    is often found in patients with _____ ; immediate   **COPD**
    treatment includes _____ .   **oxygen**

Junctional Rhythm

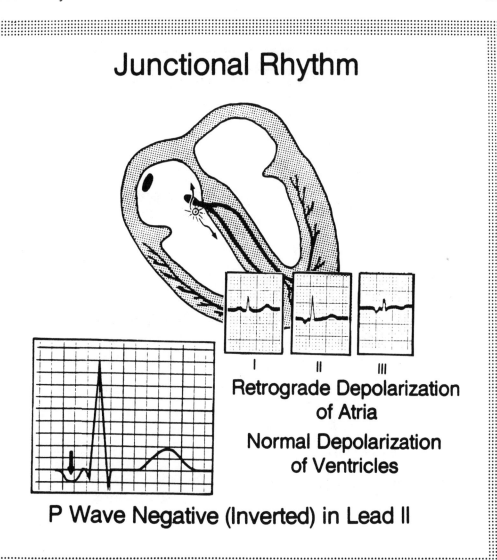

I   II   III

Retrograde Depolarization of Atria

Normal Depolarization of Ventricles

P Wave Negative (Inverted) in Lead II

When the A-V junction becomes the dominant pacemaker, the single impulse originating in the A-V junction spreads in *two* directions. The ventricles are depolarized normally, since the impulse spreads through the bundle of His to the bundle branches and then to the Purkinje network, leading to ventricular depolarization. The QRS complexes, therefore, are normal. The atria, however, are depolarized in a manner opposite that of normal. This is known as *retrograde* atrial depolarization. This retrograde atrial depolarization is reflected electrocardiographically by a *negative* (downward, inverted) P wave in leads II, III, and aVF. Normal depolarization progressing from above downward is *antegrade* depolarization. The ventricles are depolarized *antegradely* (normally). Junctional rhythm refers to a rhythm originating within the A-V junction.

In junctional rhythm:

the atria are depolarized _____ while the   retrogradely
ventricles are depolarized _____ , that is,   antegradely
normally.

the retrograde atrial depolarization is represented
electrocardiographically by a(n) _____   negative (inverted)
P wave in leads II, III, and aVF.

Junctional Rhythm
P Waves

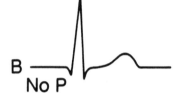

A   P↓   Atria Depolarized
             Before Ventricles

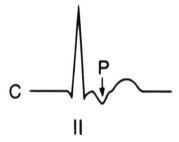

B — No P   Simultaneous
             Depolarization of
             Atria and Ventricles

C   P   Ventricles Depolarized
           Before Atria

II

The position of the P wave depends on whether:

A. The atria are depolarized _____ the ventricles. The P   before
   wave is inverted in lead II with a short (0.12 sec. or less) P-R
   interval.

B. The atria and ventricles are depolarized _____ . The P   simultaneously
   wave is then hidden within the QRS complex and is not
   visible on the electrocardiogram.

C. The atria are depolarized _____ the ventricles. The P   after
   wave is then inverted in lead II, following the QRS complex.
An additional possibility exists, as illustrated on page 221.

> The ladder diagrams of the three examples shown above are illustrated on page 383.

Junctional Rhythm
P Waves

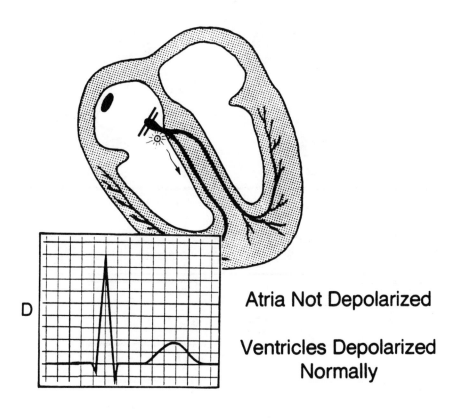

Atria Not Depolarized

Ventricles Depolarized
Normally

D

D. When no P waves are visible, a fourth possibility exists. The atria are not depolarized because retrograde conduction is blocked. The QRS complexes are normal, with normal ventricular depolarization. This possibility is illustrated on the next page.

In junctional rhythm:

when no P waves are seen, the atria and ventricles are either depolarized _____ , or the atrial depolarization is _____ .

simultaneously
blocked

when the P waves are visible before the QRS complexes, the P-R interval is usually _____ sec. or less.

0.12

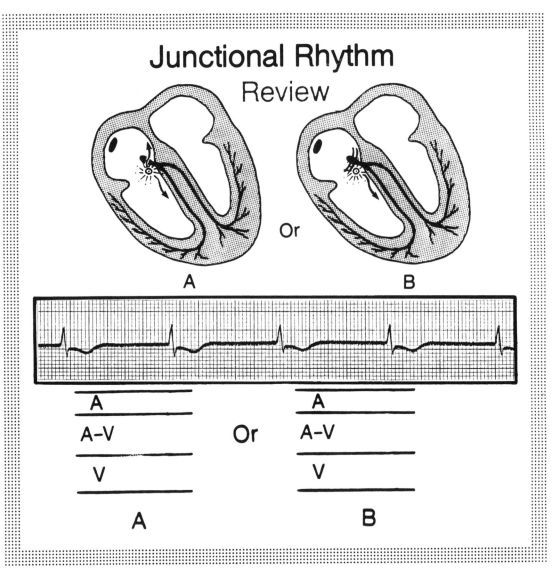

Junctional Rhythm
Review

Review:

When no P waves are present in junctional rhythm, two possibilities exist. Either the atria and ventricles are depolarized simultaneously (A), or there is retrograde block and the atria are not depolarized (B). After reviewing ladder diagrams, complete the ladder diagrams of the two possibilities cited above.

Answer:

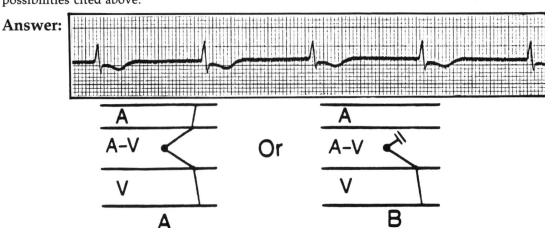

Premature Junctional Contraction (PJC)

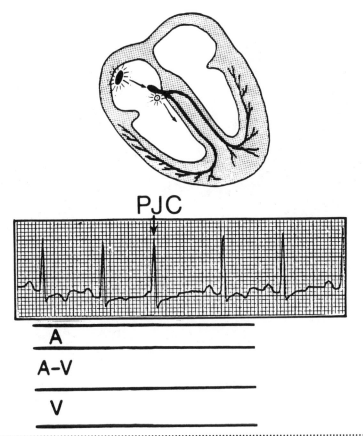

Premature junctional beats are seen when the A-V junction propagates an impulse before the next normal beat is due. In the illustration above, the PJC is seen shortly after the onset of the sinus P wave and interrupts the sinus rhythm. Complete the ladder diagram (including the cycles before and after the PJC).

Answer:

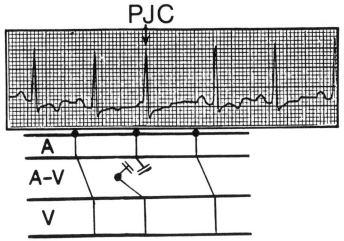

Junctional Tachycardia

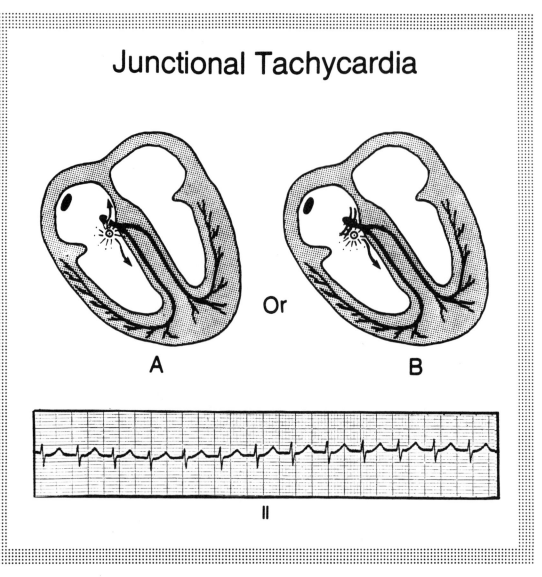

A   Or   B

II

As seen earlier, when no P waves are present with a dominant junctional pacemaker, two possibilities exist. Either the atria and ventricles are depolarized simultaneously (A), or there is retrograde block and the atria are not depolarized (B). Junctional rhythm with a rapid rate may be seen in patients with digitalis toxicity and myocardial infarction (see accelerated junctional rhythm, page 225).

In A-V junctional tachycardia the heart rate is
usually _____ to _____ per min.   100 170

Junctional rhythm with a rapid rate may be seen in
patients with _____ _____   digitalis toxicity
and _____ _____ .   myocardial infarction

Accelerated Junctional Rhythm

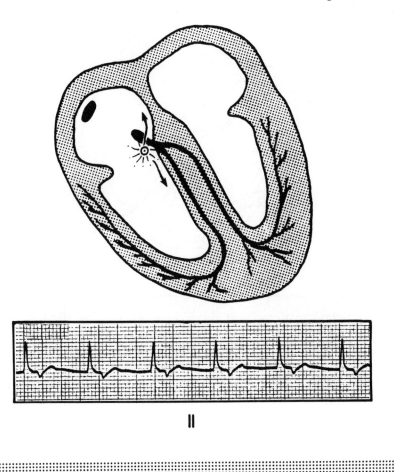

II

The inherent rate of the junctional pacemaker is 40 to 60 per min. In accelerated junctional rhythm (AJR) the rate exceeds 60 per min. (as seen in this example, at 88 per min.). Note the inverted (retrograde) P waves following the QRS complexes.

The inherent rate of the junctional pacemaker is _____ to _____ per   40 60
min.

In accelerated junctional rhythm the rate exceeds _____ per min.   60

Wandering Pacemaker

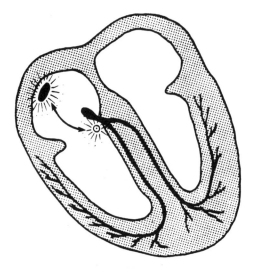

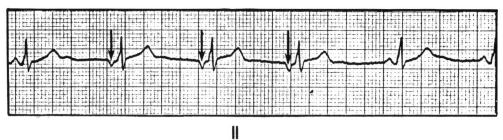

II

When pacemaker dominance is shared by more than one pacemaker, P waves of varying configurations result. This is known as a *wandering pacemaker.* Here pacemaker dominance is shared by the S-A node and the A-V junction. Notice the shift in atrial morphology (variation in P wave polarity). Following a sinus beat, there are three junctional beats (arrows) followed by the two sinus beats. Both the S-A node and the A-V junction have a P-R interval of 0.12 sec., the lower limit for the S-A node and the upper limit for the A-V junction.

**When atrial morphology shifts between two pacemakers,
the phenomenon is known
as _____ _____ .**   wandering pacemaker

**In this electrocardiogram the pacemaker shifts between
the _____ _____ and**   S-A node
the _____ _____ .   A-V junction

Junctional Escape Rhythm

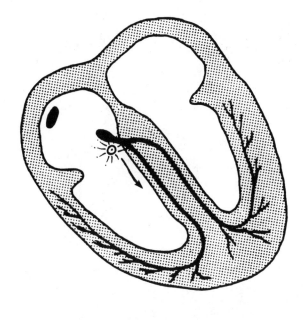

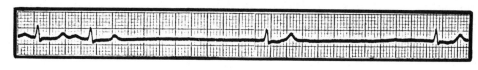

With the *arrest of the S-A node* (see page 211), a long pause follows. The beat following this pause is known as an *escape* beat, usually from a lower pacemaker, often the A-V junction, as above. If the pacemaker originating the escape beat remains the dominant one, the rhythm may then be called an *escape* or *safety rhythm,* because it may represent the only remaining pacemaker.

The junctional beat following the sinus arrest is a(n) _____ beat.   escape

An escape rhythm is often called a(n) _____ rhythm; it may   safety
represent the only remaining pacemaker.

Supraventricular Tachycardia

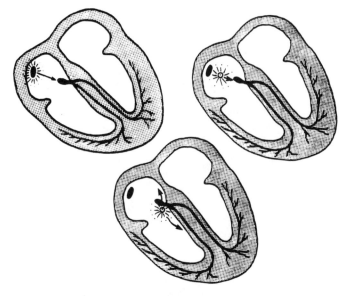

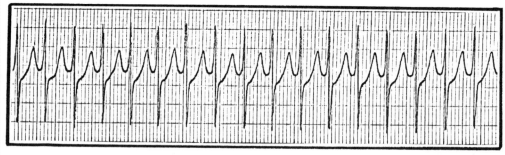

Often the P waves, because of the rate (188 above), cannot be clearly delineated to establish the diagnosis as sinus, atrial, or junctional tachycardia. Such a tachycardia is frequently classified under the overall category of *supraventricular tachycardia,* originating *above* the ventricles. The normal QRS interval (0.1 sec. or less) identifies a supraventricular pacemaker.

Supraventricular tachycardia includes _____ ,   sinus
_____ and _____ tachycardia.   atrial junctional

A normal QRS interval (0.1 sec. or less) identifies
a _____ pacemaker.   supraventricular

Ventricular Rhythm

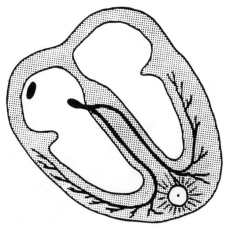

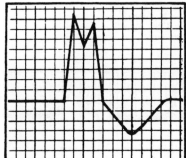

Abnormal Depolarization
of Ventricles

Atria May or May Not
Be Depolarized
Retrogradely

QRS Interval Wide,
Greater Than 0.1 sec.

An impulse originating in the *ventricles* follows an abnormal pathway of conduction and cannot depolarize the ventricles within 0.1 sec. or less. In a ventricular rhythm the QRS complex is, therefore, abnormally wide, greater than 0.1 sec., and frequently greater than 0.12 sec. (three small boxes). The QRS complex is not only wide but also often bizarre in appearance. The T wave is generally opposite the QRS in orientation. Above we have a positive QRS complex, wide and bizarre, with a negative T wave.

In a ventricular rhythm:
the QRS complex is abnormally _____ .   **wide**

accompanying the wide QRS complex
are _____abnormalities.   **repolarization**

Idioventricular Rhythm

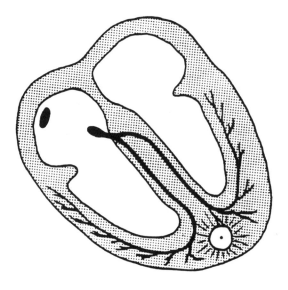

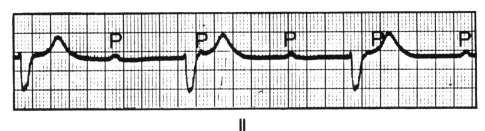

II

The inherent rate of the ventricular pacemaker is 20 to 40 per min. The above ventricular rate is 33 per min., whereas the atrial rate is 62 per min. With abnormal ventricular depolarization, the ventricular pacemaker is not as efficient as the supraventricular pacemakers. It is the lowest of the series of pacemakers and may become dominant when the higher pacemakers have failed. It may be an "escape" or "safety" rhythm and should not be suppressed.

The inherent rate of the ventricular pacemaker is _____   20
to _____ per min.   40

The ventricular rhythm may represent a(n) _____ or   escape
a(n) _____ rhythm.   safety

Premature Ventricular Contraction (PVC)

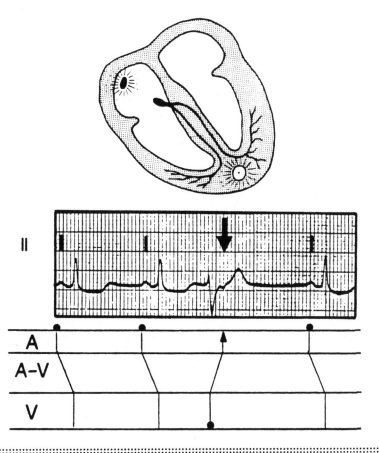

A *premature ventricular contraction (PVC)* is seen when an impulse is propagated from a ventricular focus before the next normal beat is due. The QRS complex is commonly widened and not preceded by a P wave. There may be retrograde activation of the atria following a PVC when the ventricular impulse succeeds in penetrating the conduction system all the way to the atria, producing a retrograde P wave (large arrow, above), or the sinus P waves may continue (as illustrated on page 232). The ladder diagram illustrates the origin of the PVC within the ventricles, with retrograde depolarization of the atria.

A _____ is seen when an impulse is propagated   PVC
from a ventricular focus before the next normal beat is
due.

There may be _____ _____ of the   retrograde depolarization
atria following a PVC.

Premature Ventricular Contractions
Full Compensatory Pause

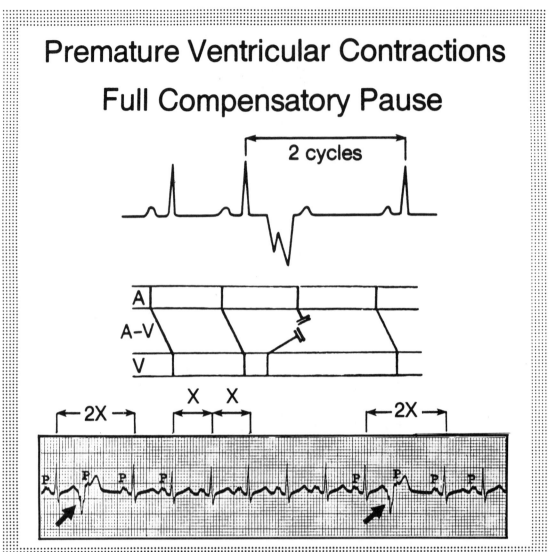

A PVC (large arrows above point to two PVCs) is frequently identified by the accompanying *compensatory pause.* When the PVC conducts retrogradely into the conduction system, the next sinus P wave finds the conduction system fully refractory, and is therefore not conducted (see page 213). The *following* sinus beat conducts normally. The R-R interval surrounding the PVC is therefore precisely equal to *two* sinus cycle lengths in a *full* compensatory pause. The ladder diagram illustrates the electrocardiographic events.

A PVC is frequently accompanied by
a(n) _____ _____ .   compensatory pause

In a full compensatory pause the interval between the QRS
complex preceding the PVC and the QRS complex following
the PVC is _____ that of the regular cycle length.   2X

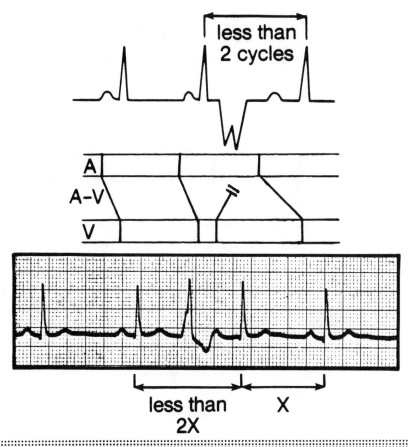

Premature Ventricular Contraction
Partial Compensatory Pause

At times, the interval between the QRS complex preceding the PVC and the QRS complex following the PVC is less than twice that of the regular cycle interval. This is a *partial compensatory pause*, occurring when the PVC conducts retrogradely into the *partially* recovered conduction system. The next sinus P wave is therefore conducted, but with an *increased P-R interval*, so that the R-R interval surrounding the PVC is equal to *between* one and two sinus cycle lengths. The ladder diagram illustrates the events leading to a partial compensatory pause.

A(n) _____ _____   partial compensatory
_____ occurs when the interval between the QRS   pause
complex preceding the PVC and the QRS complex following
the PVC is less than twice that of the regular cycle length.

When a partial compensatory pause occurs the P-R
interval of the beat following the PVC is
often _____ .   prolonged

> See page 384 for discussion of concealed conduction, explaining the findings in this electrocardiogram.

Premature Ventricular Contraction
No Pause

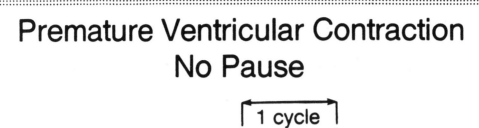

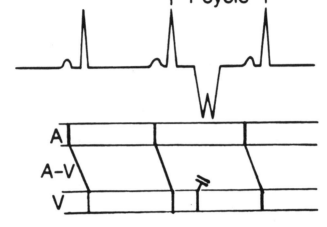

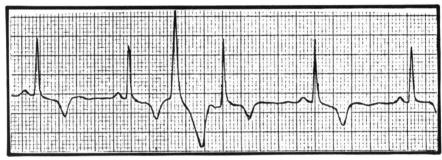

Less frequently, a PVC occurs without any pause. When the PVC barely penetrates the A-V conduction system, the next sinus P wave encounters no delay, and thus conducts normally. The PVC therefore falls precisely within one sinus cycle R-R interval. When a PVC is present between two consecutively conducted sinus beats, it is also known as an *interpolated* PVC.

When a PVC barely penetrates the A-V conduction system,
the next sinus P wave encounters no delay and there is
no _____ _____ .   compensatory pause

When a PVC is present between two consecutively conducted
sinus beats, it is also known as a(n) _____   interpolated
PVC.

Premature Ventricular Contraction
Unifocal

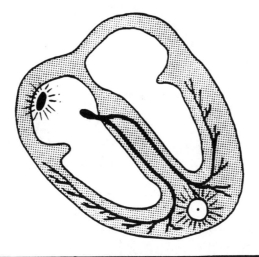

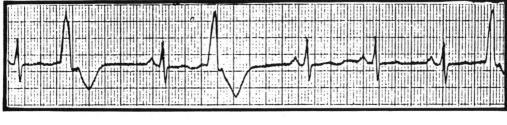

When all the PVCs originate in one focus (unifocal), they are alike in configuration in any given lead. Note the relationship of each of the three PVCs to the preceding QRS complex. The distance between the preceding QRS complex and each PVC is identical. This is known as "fixed coupling" and is seen commonly.

When all the PVCs in a given lead are alike, they are _____PVCs.

unifocal

There is _____ _____ when the distance between the preceding QRS complex and each PVC is identical.

fixed coupling

Premature Ventricular Contractions
Multifocal

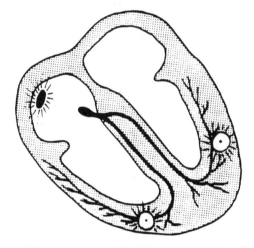

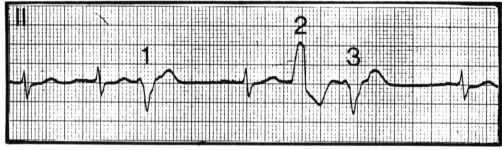

The three PVCs above originate in two foci. PVC 2 is different in configuration from PVCs 1 and 3. When PVCs originate in more than one focus, they are known as multifocal PVCs. The term "multiform" (or multiforme) has been recommended by some, since research has shown that PVCs of more than one configuration may originate in one focus.

When PVCs originate in more than one focus, they
are _____PVCs.   multifocal

The term _____ (or _____) has   multiform multiforme
been recommended because PVCs of more than one
configuration may originate in one focus.

Premature Ventricular Contractions

Couplets

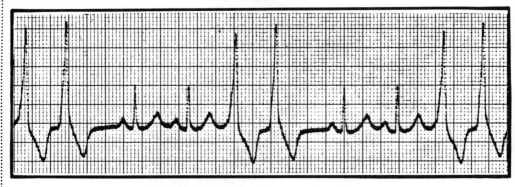

Salvo

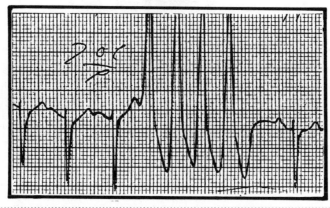

A *couplet* refers to two closely coupled PVCs in a row. A couplet should not be confused with the term coupling, which refers to the relationship of the PVC to the previous normal beat (see pages 235 and 238).

A *salvo* is a run of three or more ventricular ectopic beats in a row. By definition, this is a burst of ventricular tachycardia.

Two closely coupled PVCs in a row are a _____ . couplet

Three or more ectopic ventricular beats in a row are a _____ . salvo

Premature Ventricular Contractions
Bigeminy

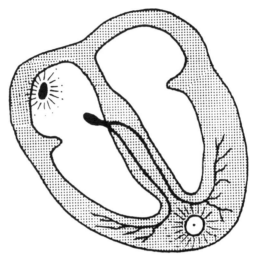

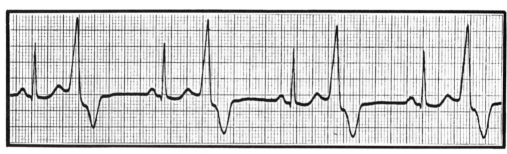

Bigeminy describes the heart beating in groups of two. In this patient each normal beat is followed by a PVC and is separated from the next group by a pause. Trigeminy refers to heart beats in groups of three. The terms bigeminy and trigeminy do not reveal the components of the group; these must be described. In this case the true sinus rate is not known. The rate could be 37 or 74 per min. If the latter is true, the nonconducted P waves are hidden within the ectopic complexes. As seen on page 235, the distance between the preceding QRS complex and each PVC is identical (fixed coupling).

_____ refers to heartbeats in groups of two.   **Bigeminy**

The terms "bigeminy" and "trigeminy" _____ _____ reveal the   **do not**
components of the group.

> See page 385 for definition of the "rule of bigeminy."

Premature Ventricular Contractions "R-on-T" Phenomenon

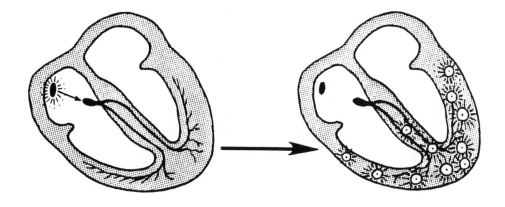

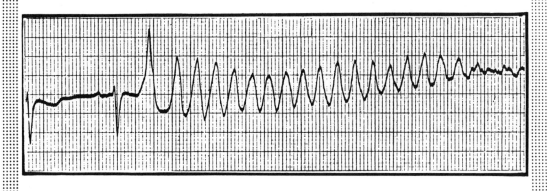

The "R-on-T" phenomenon refers to the occurrence of a premature beat on or near the peak of the T wave of the preceding beat. On page 213 we differentiated between the absolute and relative refractory periods. The peak of the T wave is a *vulnerable* period, with the ability of a premature beat to initiate ventricular tachycardia, flutter or fibrillation. The study of these arrhythmias is found on the next few pages. Here we see an "R-on-T" setting off a catastrophic arrhythmia.

A PVC occurring on or near the peak of the T wave of the previous
beat is known as the _____ ____ _____ phenomenon.   "R-on-T"

The peak of the T wave is a(n) _____ period.   vulnerable

Ventricular Tachycardia
(Sustained)

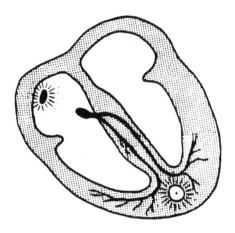

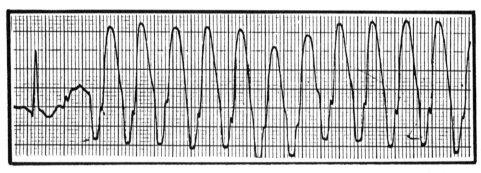

Once started, *ventricular tachycardia* may be sustained until terminated spontaneously, by medication, or by electrical cardioversion, or it may be intermittent. The QRS complexes are widened and bizarre, and the rate is usually from 150 to 250 per min. The rhythm may be regular or slightly irregular. Atrial activity, dissociated from ventricular activity, may not be affected.

In ventricular tachycardia:
    the heart rate is usually _____ to _____ per min.   **250 350**

    atrial activity, dissociated from ventricular
    activity, _____ _____ be affected.   **may not**

> See pages 386 to 389 for a discussion of fusion and parasystole in the understanding of ventricular rhythms.

Ventricular Tachycardia
(Intermittent)

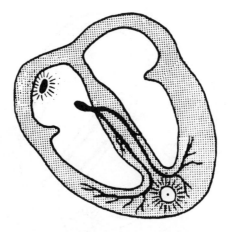

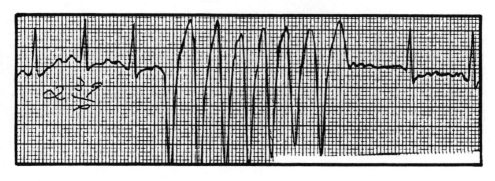

As noted on the previous page, ventricular tachycardia may be sustained or intermittent.

Ventricular tachycardia may be _____   sustained
or _____ .   intermittent

The QRS complexes in ventricular tachycardia
are _____ and _____ .   wide bizarre

Ventricular Tachycardia
(Torsades de Pointes)

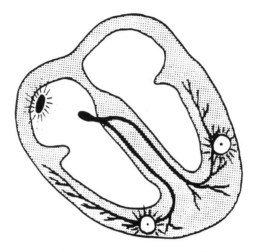

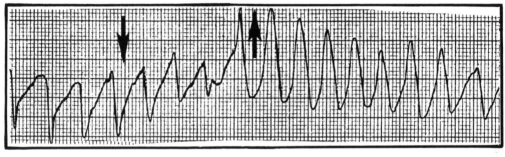

Ventricular tachycardia may be unifocal or multifocal ("polymorphic"). In a given lead there may be beats of one polarity followed by beats of the opposite polarity separated by beats of an intermediate form. This is known as torsades de pointes (twistings of the points).

Ventricular tachycardia may be ———————————— or ———————————— .

unifocal
multifocal

In ventricular tachycardia there may be QRS complexes of one polarity followed by QRS complexes of the opposite polarity separated by QRS complexes of an intermediate form; this is known as ———————— ——— ———————— .

torsades de pointes

Accelerated Idioventricular Rhythm (AIVR)

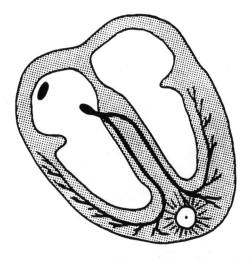

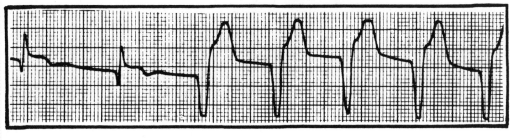

Normally, the latent ventricular pacemaker has an "escape" rate of 40 per min. or less. The *accelerated* idioventricular rhythm (AIVR) controls the heart at a rate from 40 to 150 (usually 60 to 130) per min. This ectopic rhythm may be an "escape" or "safety" rhythm when the higher pacemakers begin to slow down or fail completely. It is commonly seen in patients with myocardial infarction. It very rarely progresses to a serious tachycardia and should not be suppressed.

When the idioventricular pacemaker is accelerated to a rate of 40 to 150 per min. it is known as _____ .   **AIVR**

AIVR may be a(n) _____ __ _____ rhythm and should not be suppressed.   **escape or safety**

> The subject of the wide QRS complex with a *supraventricular* pacemaker is explained and illustrated on pages 390 to 396, including LBBB and RBBB, aberrant ventricular conduction and the Ashman phenomenon, bundle of His studies, and pre-excitation (the W-P-W and L-G-L syndromes).

Ventricular Flutter

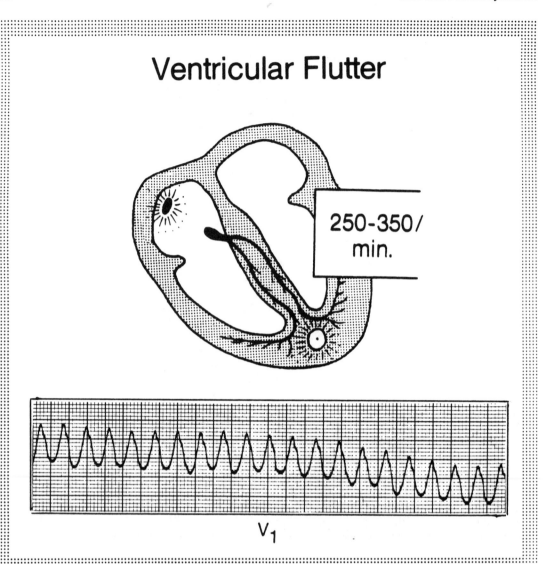

250-350/min.

V_1

In *ventricular flutter*, undulating waves are seen rising and falling. This rhythm is often an intermediary stage between ventricular tachycardia and ventricular fibrillation. The rate is usually between 250 and 350 per min. When the ventricular rate is at this level, the patient is acutely ill and the pulse may be imperceptible. This rhythm requires immediate interruption to sustain life. Atrial activity may be unaffected. The rhythm is usually short-lived, deteriorating into ventricular fibrillation within a very short time.

In ventricular flutter the ventricular rate is _____   250
to _____ per min.   350

Ventricular flutter may deteriorate
into _____ _____within a   ventricular fibrillation.
very short time.

Ventricular Fibrillation

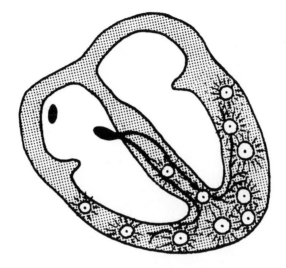

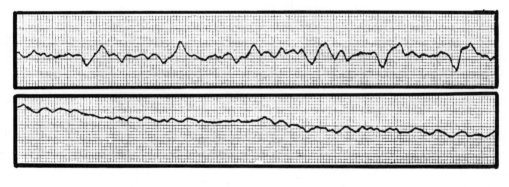

Multiple, disorganized contractions of the ventricles characterize *ventricular fibrillation* and represent *cardiac arrest*. It may be of sudden onset or may follow ventricular premature contractions, ventricular tachycardia and ventricular flutter. The immediate institution of cardiopulmonary resuscitation while waiting for electrical defibrillation may be lifesaving.

**Multiple, disorganized contractions of the ventricles
characterize** _____ _____ .   **ventricular fibrillation**

**Ventricular fibrillation
represents** _____ _____ .   **cardiac arrest**

Practice
ECG Analysis

Practice
ECG Analysis

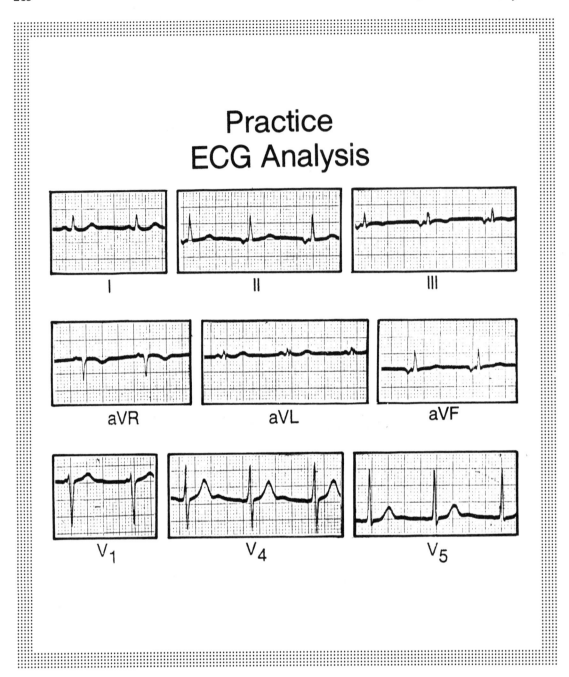

The patient is an asymptomatic 35-year-old man.

Analysis:

ECG ANALYSIS

1. Rhythm and rate
   Rhythm: A-V junctional
   Rate: 75/min.
   P-R interval: 0.1 sec.
   P waves are negative in leads II, III, and aVF
2. QRS complex
   Duration: 0.08 sec.
   Axis: +60°
3. Ventricular repolarization
   S-T segment: neither significantly elevated nor depressed
   T wave: QRS-T angle normal
   Q-T interval: 0.35 sec.

Impression and Comment

A-V junctional rhythm

The A-V junction may be the dominant pacemaker congenitally or may share dominance with the S-A node throughout life. Because the intrinsic A-V junctional rate is 40 to 60 per min., a rate of 85 per min. is really an acceleration of the A-V junction. In an A-V junctional rhythm the P waves are usually upright in lead I but may be transitional or slightly negative and negative in leads II and III; they may come before, during or after the QRS complex. When the P wave precedes the QRS complex, the P-R interval is usually short, up to 0.12 sec. If the atria are not depolarized, a P wave will not be present. The QRS complexes are generally normal, because ventricular depolarization proceeds normally.

Practice
ECG Analysis

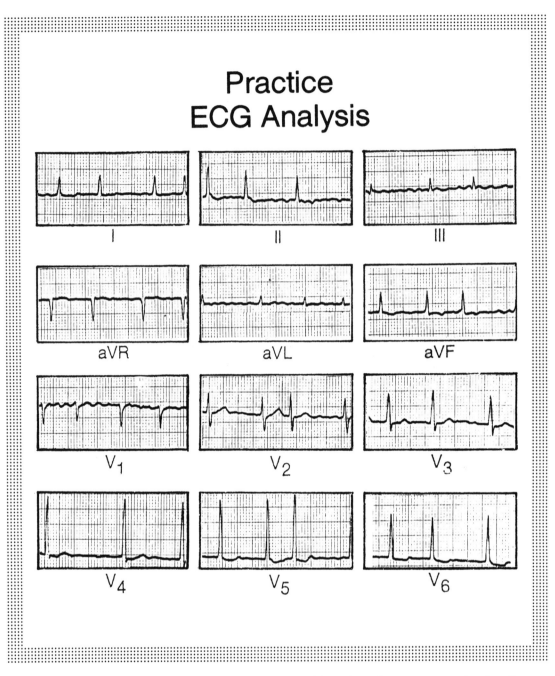

The patient is a 78-year-old man with shortness of breath and angina pectoris who discontinued his digitalis one week earlier.

Analysis:

ECG ANALYSIS

1. Rhythm and rate
   Rhythm: atrial fibrillation
   Rate: 95/min., average
   No P waves are present, only fibrillatory atrial waves
2. QRS complex
   Duration: 0.08 sec.
   Axis: $+45°$
3. Ventricular repolarization
   S-T segment: depressed, leads II, aVF, V_5, and V_6
   T wave: low throughout, with a wide QRS-T angle
   Q-T interval: 0.30 sec.

Impression and Comment

Atrial fibrillation with moderate ventricular response
Ventricular repolarization (ST-T) abnormalities

We see the typical irregularly irregular ventricular response that usually accompanies atrial fibrillation. The ventricular rate depends on how many of 350 to 600 atrial impulses are conducted to the ventricles. One of the actions of digitalis is to increase the block at the A-V node, thereby slowing the ventricular rate. Although the patient had not been taking digitalis for one week, some "digitalis effects" may still be observed with the rounding of the S-T segment depression, best seen in lead V_5. The ST-T abnormalities may be caused predominantly by the myocardial ischemia associated with the patient's coronary heart disease.

Additional Electrocardiograms for Practice and Review

As mentioned in the preface, in this era of high technology, most of the electrocardiograms in this section have been recorded on the multichannel system in common use in most hospitals. These electrocardiograms are mounted to preserve the simultaneous recording of the various leads. They have been altered only to fit the page.

Practice
ECG Analysis

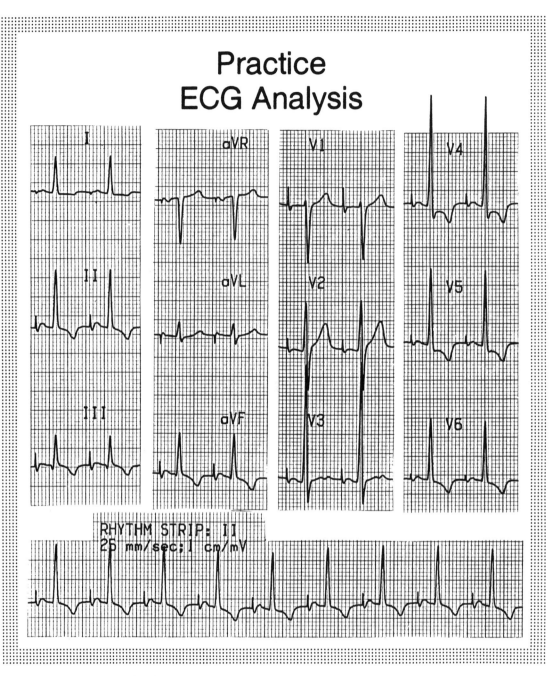

Practice ECG Analysis 1.

The patient is a 68-year-old man with a history of hypertension controlled on medication. In the recent 2 weeks he had three episodes of "almost fainting."

Analysis:

ECG ANALYSIS 1

1. Rhythm and rate
   Rhythm: artificial atrial pacing
   Rate: 100/min.
   P-R Interval: 0.2 sec. interval between atrial pacemaker and onset of ventricular depolarization
2. QRS complex
   Duration: 0.08 sec.
   Axis: +50°
3. Ventricular repolarization
   S-T segment: depressed in leads II, aVF, and V_4 to V_6
   T wave: inverted in leads I, II, III, aVF, and V_4 to V_6, QRS-T angle wide
4. Q-T interval: 0.31 sec.

Impression and Comment

Artificial atrial pacing
Left ventricular hypertrophy
Ventricular repolarization abnormalities

This patient, with a many-year history of controlled hypertension, developed a "sick sinus" syndrome with several episodes of "near fainting." Electrophysiologic studies confirmed good A-V conduction, and artificial atrial pacing eliminated these recent symptoms. Although the commonly accepted criteria for left ventricular hypertrophy (LVH) are not met here, the findings of Roberts and Day are seen (see page 364). These investigators analyzed findings in patients with aortic insufficiency and added the following criterion for left ventricular hypertrophy: Total QRS amplitude in all 12 electrocardiographic leads >175 mm. Echocardiographic evaluation confirmed LVH in this patient.

Practice ECG Analysis

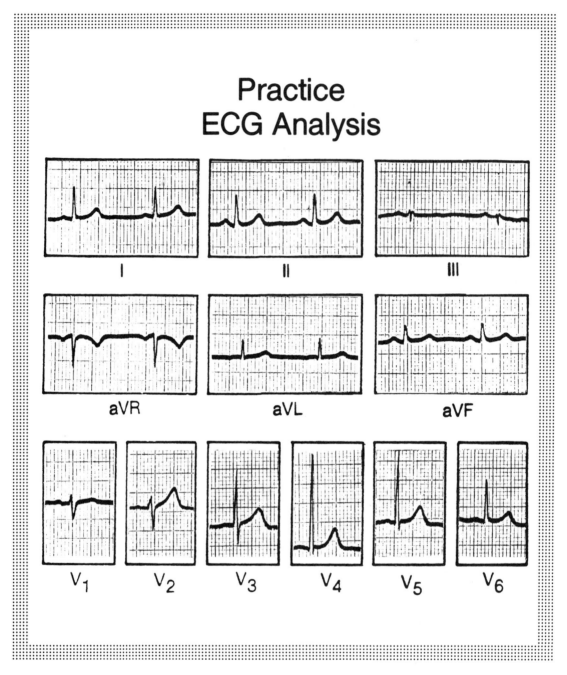

Practice ECG Analysis 2.

The patient is a healthy 46-year-old man.

Analysis:

ECG ANALYSIS 2

1. Rhythm and rate
   Rhythm: sinus
   Rate: 67/min.
   P-R interval: 0.14 sec.
2. QRS complex
   Duration: 0.08 sec.
   Axis: +30°
3. Ventricular repolarization
   S-T segment: neither significantly elevated nor depressed
   T wave: QRS-T angle normal
4. Q-T interval: 0.36 sec.

Impression and Comment

Normal electrocardiogram

Practice
ECG Analysis

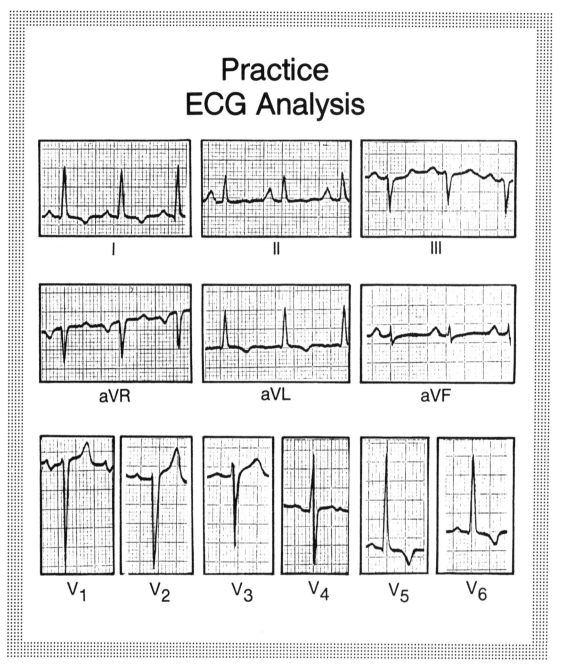

Practice ECG Analysis 3.

The patient is a 78 year old man with a long history of hypertension and congestive heart failure. Blood pressure at present is 130/80 mm. Hg.

Analysis:

ECG ANALYSIS 3

1. Rhythm and rate
   Rhythm: sinus
   Rate: 92/min.
   P-R interval: 0.18 sec.
   Tall, peaked P waves, leads II and aVF; biphasic P waves, lead V_1, overall size, 3 mm.
2. QRS complex
   Duration: 0.09 sec.
   Axis: 0°
   $S_{V1} + R_{V5} = 55$ mm.
3. Ventricular repolarization
   S-T segment: neither significantly elevated nor depressed
   T wave: very wide QRS-T angle
4. Q-T interval: 0.32 sec.

Impression and Comment

Sinus rhythm
Right and left atrial enlargement
Right and left ventricular hypertrophy
Ventricular repolarization abnormalities

Right atrial enlargement is reflected in the tall peaked P waves, seen especially well in lead II. Right atrial enlargement is good *presumptive* evidence of right ventricular hypertrophy because it rarely occurs without right ventricular hypertrophy. Direct electrocardiographic evidence of right ventricular hypertrophy is often obscured by the dominant left ventricle.

Left atrial enlargement is best seen in lead V_1. The normal P wave in lead V_1 is usually 1 to 2 mm. in magnitude. Here we have a P wave of 3 mm., with the second half of the biphasic P wave significantly negative. The criteria for left ventricular hypertrophy include the great magnitude of the QRS complexes in addition to the associated repolarization abnormalities.

This elderly patient had a very large heart with all four chambers enlarged.

Practice
ECG Analysis

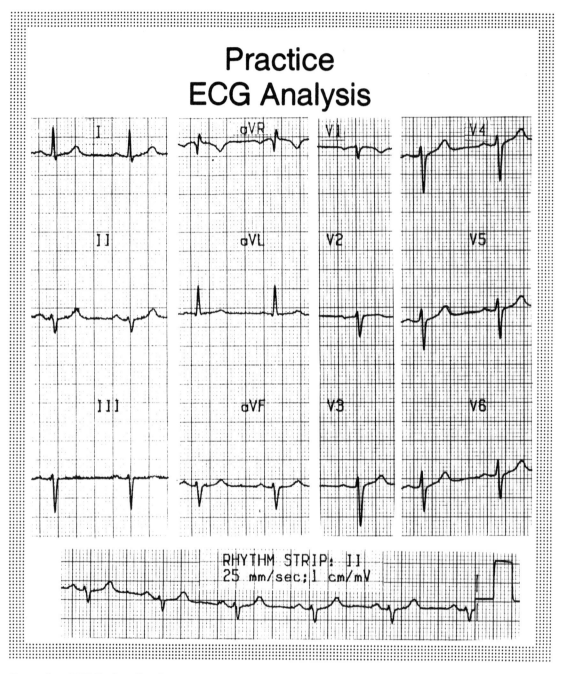

Practice ECG Analysis 4.

The patient is a 76-year-old asymptomatic man.

Analysis:

ECG ANALYSIS 4

1. Rhythm and rate
    Rhythm: sinus
    Rate: 72/min.
    P-R interval: 0.16 sec.
2. QRS complex
    Duration: 0.08 sec.
    Axis: $-60°$
    Marked clockwise rotation
3. Ventricular repolarization
    S-T segment: neither significantly elevated nor depressed
    T wave: wide QRS-T angle
4. Q-T interval: 0.36 sec.

Impression and Comment

Sinus rhythm

Marked left axis deviation of the mean QRS vector (left anterior hemiblock)

Marked clockwise rotation

Ventricular repolarization abnormalities (wide QRS-T angle)

   Although this patient is asymptomatic, it is recommended that he be checked regularly since his present electrocardiogram varies from the normal. It is important to watch for possible future changes.

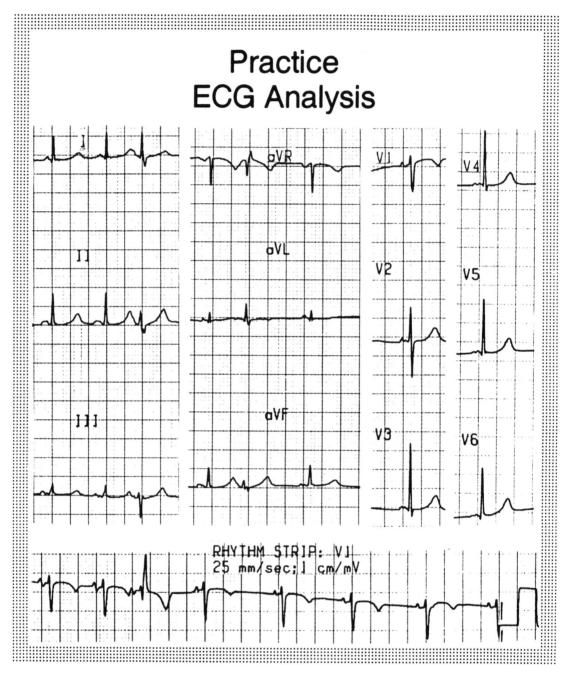

Practice ECG Analysis 5.

The patient is a 76-year-old woman with a 2-month history of palpitations.

Analysis:

ECG ANALYSIS 5

1. Rhythm and rate

    Rhythm: sinus arrhythmia with premature atrial systoles followed by aberrant ventricular conduction

    Rate: 95/min. (average)

    P-R interval: 0.12 sec. in the basic rhythm and 0.14 sec. following the premature P wave

2. QRS complex

    Duration: 0.06 sec. in basic rhythm and 0.12 sec. in aberrant beats

    Axis: $+55°$ in basic rhythm

    The aberrantly conducted beats are wide, containing an S wave in lead I and an RSR' in lead V_1, revealing a right bundle branch block pattern

3. Ventricular repolarization

    S-T segment: neither significantly elevated nor depressed

    T wave: QRS-T angle normal

    In the aberrantly conducted beats the ventricular repolarization changes are secondary to the right bundle branch block (the T waves are opposite the terminal part of the QRS complex).

4. Q-T interval: 0.36 sec. (basic rhythm) and 0.34 sec. (in the aberrantly conducted beats)

Impression and Comment

Sinus arrhythmia

Premature atrial systoles with aberrant ventricular conduction

The cause of her palpitations are the premature atrial systoles. These frequently respond to discontinuation of substances such as tobacco and caffeine.

The right bundle branch block pattern following the premature P waves represents aberrant ventricular conduction.

Cardiac evaluation revealed no other abnormalities.

Practice
ECG Analysis

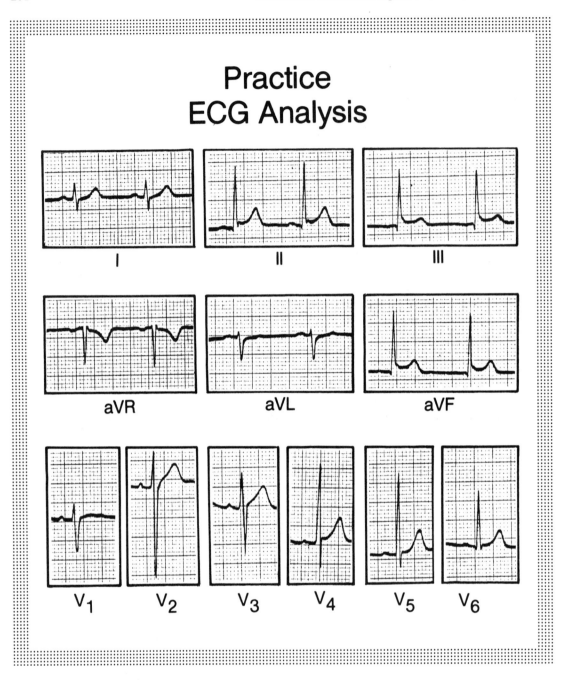

Practice ECG Analysis 6.

The patient is a healthy 18-year-old student.

Analysis:

ECG ANALYSIS 6

1. Rhythm and rate
    Rhythm: sinus
    Rate: 75/min.
    P-R interval: 0.14 sec.
2. QRS complex
    Duration: 0.08 sec.
    Axis: +85°
3. Ventricular repolarization
    S-T segment: elevated origin of the S-T segment, especially well seen on leads II, III, aVF, V_4, and V_5
    T wave: QRS-T angle normal
4. Q-T interval: 0.35 sec.

Impression and Comment

Normal electrocardiogram with early repolarization

Early repolarization is a common variant seen in normal young adults. The electrocardiogram is normal in all other respects. Of importance is the need to distinguish early repolarization from the more ominous causes of S-T segment displacement, such as pericarditis or myocardial infarction.

Practice
ECG Analysis

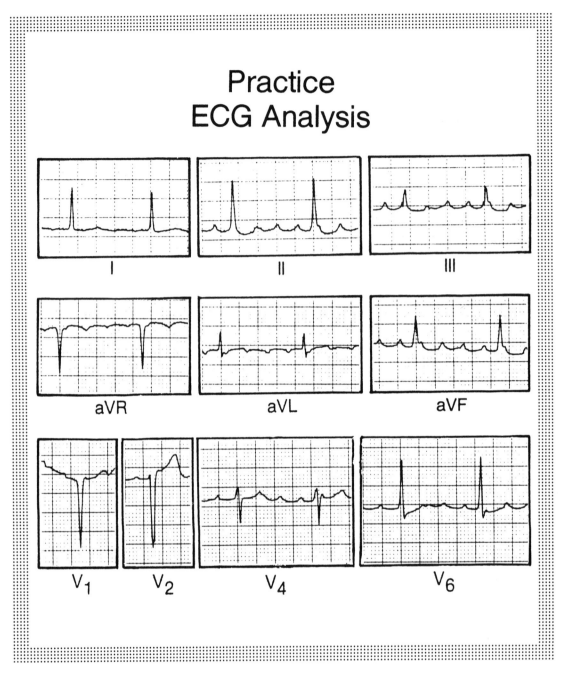

Practice ECG Analysis 7.

The patient is an adult with a history of a heart rhythm disturbance.

Analysis:

ECG ANALYSIS 7

1. Rhythm and rate
   Rhythm: atrial flutter (with a 4:1 A-V conduction ratio)
   Rate: atrial, 260/min.; ventricular, 65/min.
2. QRS complex
   Duration: 0.08 sec.
   Axis: +45°
3. Ventricular repolarization
   S-T segment: depressed and rounded, seen best in leads II, III, and aVF
   T wave: difficult to fully evaluate in the presence of flutter waves but appears low in leads I and V_6
4. Q-T interval: 0.36 sec.

Impression and Comment

Atrial flutter with a 4:1 A-V conduction ratio
Ventricular repolarization (ST-T) abnormalities (compatible with digitalis effects and/or ischemia)

With a stable 4:1 relationship between the atria and ventricles, the ventricular rate is regular at 65/min., whereas the atria are fluttering at a rate of 260/min. The rounding of the S-T segment suggests that digitalis has been used to treat this patient.

Practice
ECG Analysis

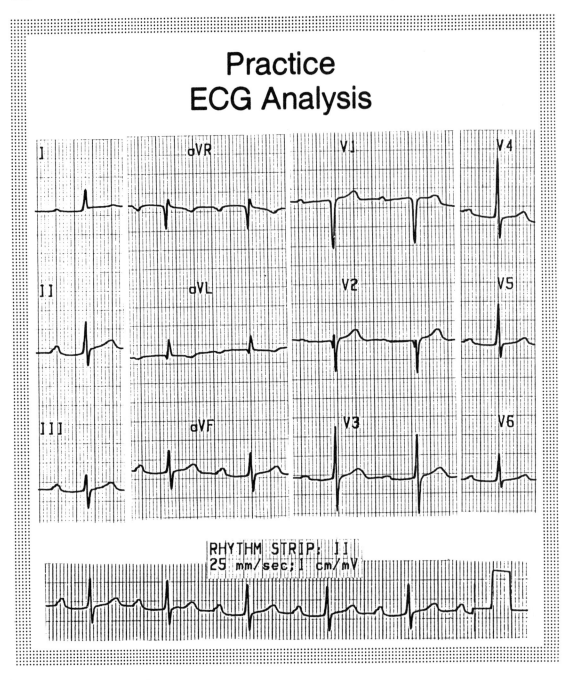

Practice ECG Analysis 8.

This patient is a 60-year-old asymptomatic man who had a heart attack 2 years earlier.

Analysis:

ECG ANALYSIS 8

1. Rhythm and rate
   Rhythm: sinus
   Rate: 68/min.
   P-R interval: 0.34 sec.
2. QRS complex
   Duration: 0.08 sec.
   Axis: $+15°$
   Significant Q waves in leads V_1 and V_2
3. Ventricular repolarization
   S-T segment: neither significantly elevated nor depressed.
   T wave: normal QRS-T angle
4. Q-T interval: 0.36 sec.

Impression and Comment

First degree A-V block
Anteroseptal myocardial infarction, old

   Although the patient is currently asymptomatic, the marked first degree A-V block must be carefully watched. If it progresses, or if a higher degree of A-V block occurs with activity, artificial pacemaker therapy may be required. Although the Q wave in lead V_2 is small, it is significant because there should not be any Q waves in the right precordial leads. The Q waves in leads V_1 and V_2 are the markers of his documented old anteroseptal myocardial infarction.

Practice
ECG Analysis

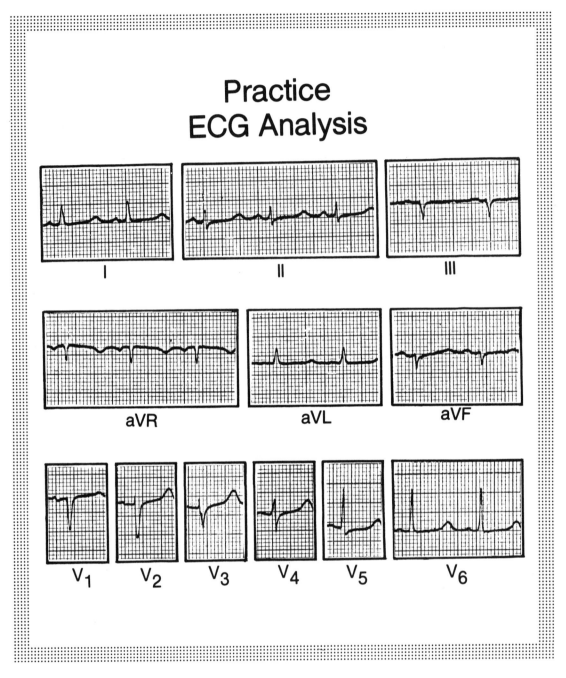

Practice ECG Analysis 9.

The patient is a 75-year-old woman with a long history of hypoparathyroidism.

Analysis:

ECG ANALYSIS 9

1. Rhythm and rate
     Rhythm: sinus
     Rate: 80/min.
     P-R interval: 0.14 sec.
2. QRS complex
     Duration: 0.08 sec.
     Axis: $-15°$
3. Ventricular repolarization
     S-T segment: neither significantly elevated nor depressed
     T wave: normal QRS-T angle
4. Q-T interval: 0.52 sec.

Impression and Comment

Sinus rhythm

Q-T interval markedly prolonged, compatible with hypocalcemia

   Marked prolongation of the Q-T interval is compatible with the hypocalcemia of hypopara-thyroidism. At this patient's heart rate of 84 per min., the Q-T interval should be approximately 0.35 sec., rather than 0.52 sec., as seen here. The relationship between the Q-T interval and the heart rate is as follows:

Heart Rate/min.	Q-T Interval set
40	0.46
60	0.39
80	0.35
100	0.31
120	0.29
140	0.26
160	0.25

Practice
ECG Analysis

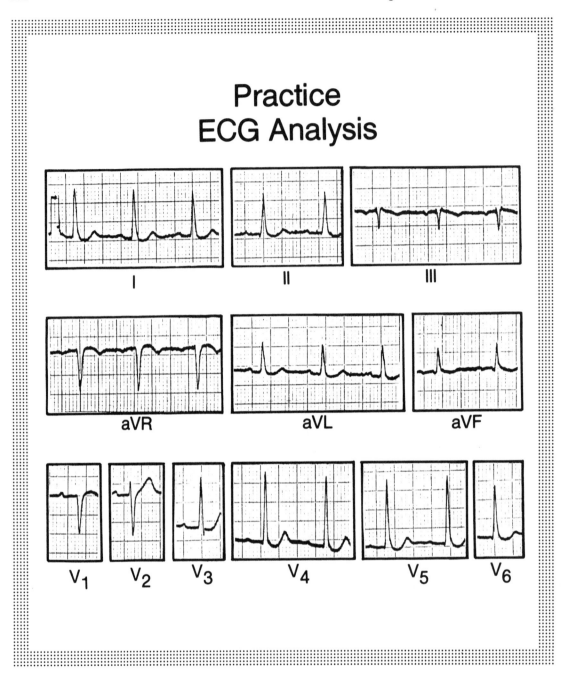

Practice ECG Analysis 10.

The patient is a 68-year-old man with long-standing congestive heart failure. He is taking digitalis and diuretics.

Analysis:

ECG ANALYSIS 10

1. Rhythm and rate
   Rhythm: sinus
   Rate: 90/min.
   P-R interval: 0.15 sec.
2. QRS complex
   Duration: 0.08 sec.
   Axis: $+15°$
3. Ventricular repolarization
   S-T segment: "paintbrush" inscription in leads I, II, aVL, V_4, V_5, and V_6
   T wave: QRS-T angle normal
4. Q-T interval: 0.32 sec.

Impression and Comment

Sinus rhythm

Ventricular repolarization alterations with "digitalis effects" on the S-T segment

The classic changes of the S-T segment caused by digitalis have been described as a "paintbrush" inscription, as if you were painting the S-T segment, with gradual widening of the paintbrush stroke. These changes have also been described as a "fist-like" depression of the S-T segment, as if you were placing a fist on the S-T segment and depressing it.

Practice ECG Analysis

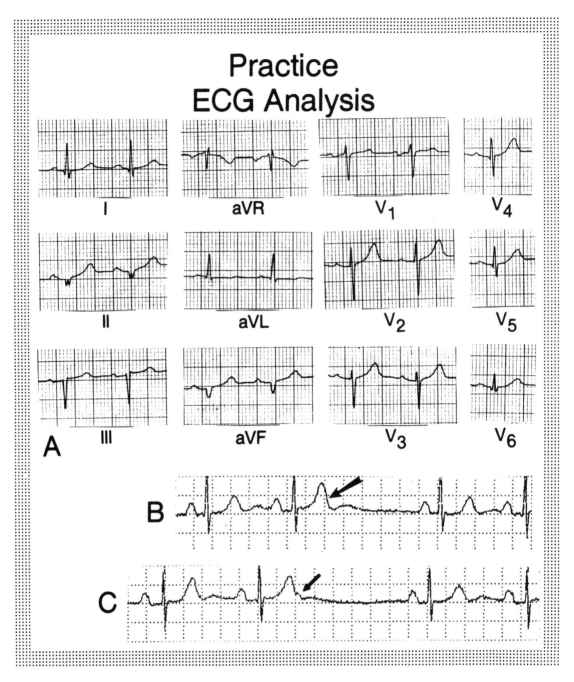

Practice ECG Analysis 11.

The patient is a 71-year-old woman with a history of episodic "skipped heart beats." She suffered a heart attack several years earlier.

Analysis:

ECG ANALYSIS 11

1. Rhythm and rate
    Rhythm: sinus
    Rate: 85/min. (ECG A), 55 to 65 (basic rate on rhythm strips B and C)
    P-R interval: 0.20 to 0.22 sec.; rhythms B and C reveal a sudden prolongation of an R-R
    interval
2. QRS complex
    Duration: 0.08 sec.
    Axis: $-40°$
    QS complexes in leads II and aVF
3. Ventricular repolarization
    S-T segment: neither significantly elevated nor depressed
    T wave: wide QRS-T angle
4. Q-T interval: 0.38 to 0.40 sec.

Impression and Comment

Sinus rhythm with premature atrial contractions (blocked)
Inferior (diaphragmatic) myocardial infarction, old
First degree A-V block (borderline)

  Although the resting electrocardiogram A does not demonstrate any rhythm disturbance, the
monitored rhythm strips reveal the "skipped beats." In B the clue to the blocked premature
atrial beat is the tall T wave (large arrow), which is the summation of the T wave of the previous
beat and the blocked P wave. In rhythm strip C the blocked P wave is seen emerging from the
T wave (small arrow).

Practice
ECG Analysis

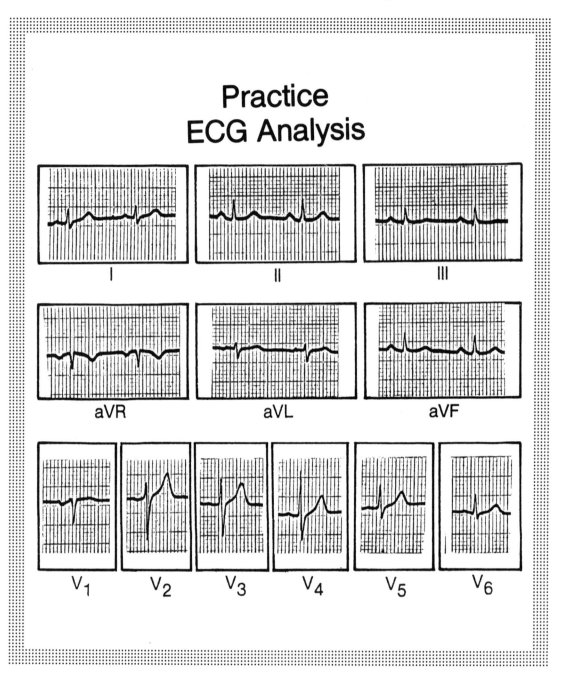

Practice ECG Analysis 12.

The patient is a 40-year-old healthy woman.

Analysis:

ECG ANALYSIS 12

1. Rhythm and rate
    Rhythm: sinus
    Rate: 80/min.
    P-R interval: 0.16 sec.
2. QRS complex
    Duration: 0.08 sec.
    Axis: 75°
3. Ventricular repolarization
    S-T segment: neither significantly elevated nor depressed
    T wave: QRS-T angle normal
4. Q-T interval: 0.35 sec.

Impression and Comment

Normal electrocardiogram

Practice
ECG Analysis

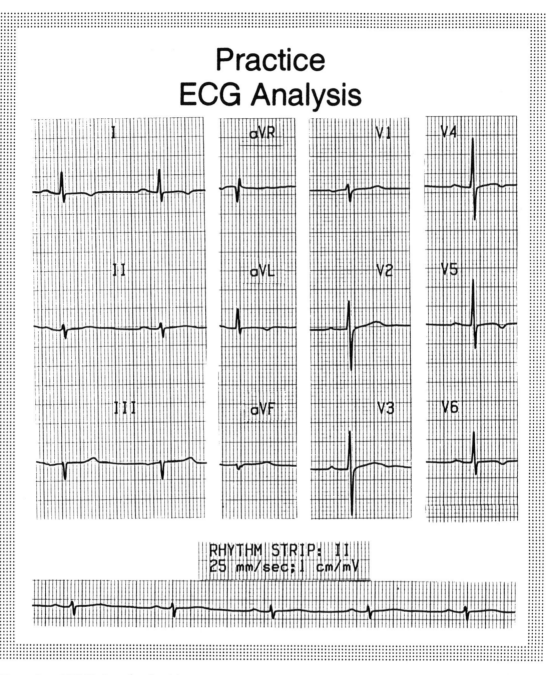

RHYTHM STRIP: II
25 mm/sec; 1 cm/mV

Practice ECG Analysis 13.

The patient is a 57-year-old man who develops shortness of breath on exertion. His daily work is sedentary.

Analysis:

ECG ANALYSIS 13

1. Rhythm and rate
     Rhythm: sinus
     Rate: 55/min.
     P-R interval: 0.20 sec.
2. QRS complex
     Duration: 0.08 sec.
     Axis: $-35°$
3. Ventricular repolarization
     S-T segment: neither significantly elevated nor depressed
     T wave: inverted in leads I, aVL, and V_4 to V_6; QRS-T angle wide
4. Q-T interval: 0.4 sec.

Impression and Comment

Sinus bradycardia

Left axis deviation of the mean QRS vector

Ventricular repolarization abnormalities, nonspecific

   Sinus bradycardia is common in an athletic person. Here, however, we have a sedentary man who becomes dyspneic on effort. In the presence of left axis deviation and ventricular repolarization abnormalities, a full cardiac evaluation is essential.

Practice
ECG Analysis

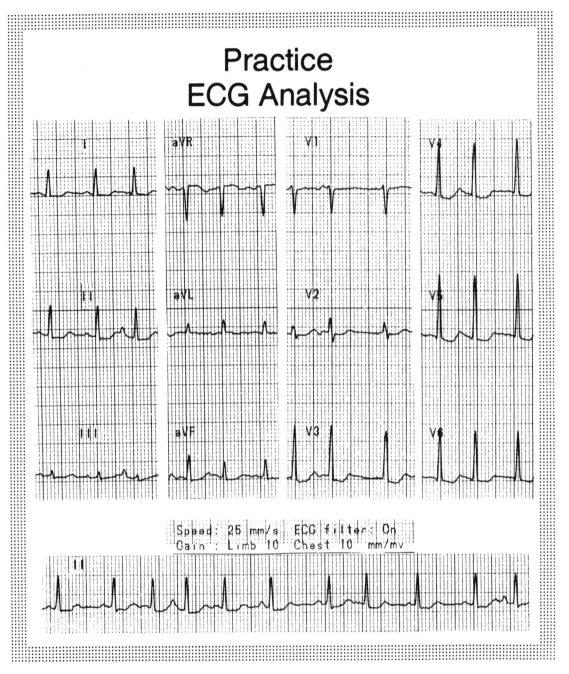

Speed: 25 mm/s   ECG filter: On
Gain : Limb 10   Chest 10   mm/mv

Practice ECG Analysis 14.

An 81-year-old woman with chronic lung disease presents with cough, shortness of breath, and palpitations.

Analysis:

ECG ANALYSIS 14

1. Rhythm and rate
    Rhythm: multifocal atrial tachycardia
    Rate: 130/min. (average)
    P-R interval: varies with the multiple foci
2. QRS complex
    Duration: 0.06 sec.
    Axis: +40°
3. Ventricular repolarization
    S-T segment: depressed in leads I, II, aVF, V_5, and V_6
    T wave: QRS-T angle within normal limits
4. Q-T interval: 0.32 sec.

Impression and Comment

Multifocal (chaotic) atrial tachycardia

Ventricular repolarization abnormalities, nonspecific

   Multifocal atrial tachycardia is most common in patients with chronic lung disease and a low Po_2, exacerbated by pulmonary infection. Oxygen therapy often promptly terminates this arrhythmia. This rhythm is sometimes mistaken for atrial fibrillation because it is also irregularly irregular and because the P waves are not distinctly seen in all the leads.

Practice
ECG Analysis

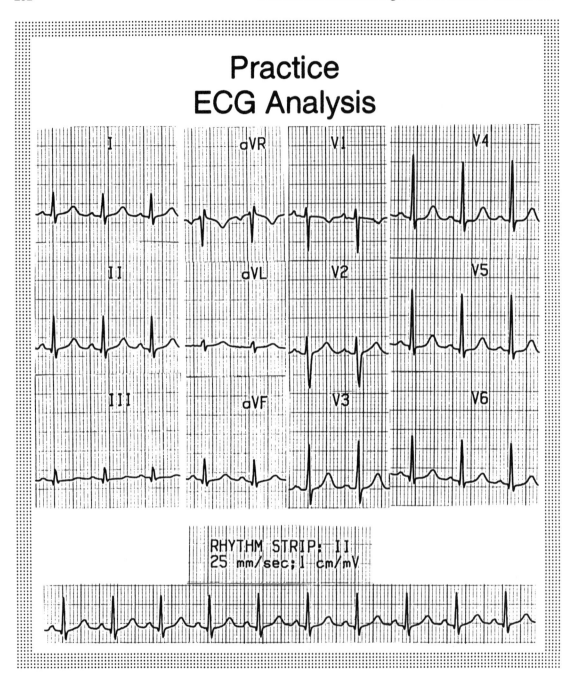

Practice ECG Analysis 15.

The patient is a 22-year-old healthy woman immediately after jogging.

Analysis:

ECG ANALYSIS 15

1. Rhythm and rate
   Rhythm: sinus
   Rate: 110/min.
   P-R interval: 0.14 sec.
2. QRS complex
   Duration: 0.08 sec.
   Axis: +60°
3. Ventricular repolarization
   S-T segment: neither significantly elevated nor depressed
   T wave: QRS-T angle normal
4. Q-T interval: 0.32 sec.

Impression and Comment

Sinus tachycardia

This electrocardiogram is normal in a 22-year-old woman after jogging.

Practice
ECG Analysis

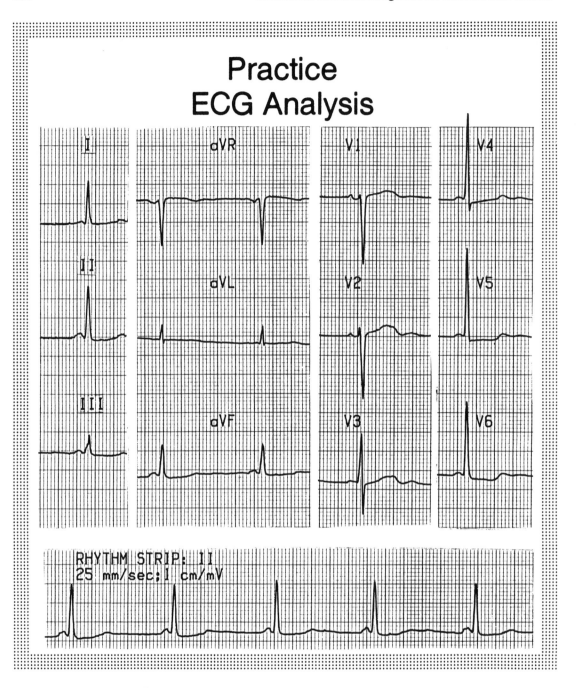

Practice ECG Analysis 16.

The patient is a 50-year-old woman with a many-year history of palpitations.

Analysis:

ECG ANALYSIS 16

1. Rhythm and rate
   Rhythm: sinus
   Rate: 55/min.
   P-R interval: 0.10 sec.
2. QRS complex
   Duration: 0.08 sec.
   Axis: $+45°$
3. Ventricular repolarization
   S-T segment: depressed, best seen in leads II, V_5, and V_6
   T wave: low, but QRS-T angle within normal limits
4. Q-T interval: 0.44 sec.

Impression and Comment

Sinus bradycardia

Short P-R interval Lown-Ganong-Levine (L-G-L) syndrome

Ventricular repolarization abnormalities, nonspecific

   The short P-R interval syndrome has been associated with various arrhythmias. This syndrome was described by Lown, Ganong, and Levine and is often called the L-G-L syndrome. Although no rhythm disturbance is seen on this electrocardiogram, the episodic rhythm disturbances associated with the short P-R interval syndrome may be responsible for her complaint of palpitations.

Practice
ECG Analysis

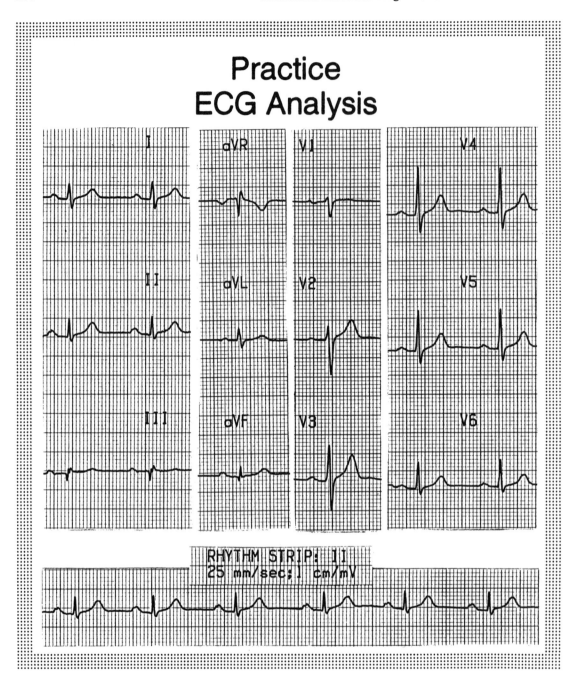

Practice ECG Analysis 17.

The patient is a 40-year-old asymptomatic man.

Analysis:

ECG ANALYSIS 17

1. Rhythm and rate
   Rhythm: sinus
   Rate: 65/min.
   P-R interval: 0.22 sec.
2. QRS complex
   Duration: 0.08 sec.
   Axis: $+15°$
3. Ventricular repolarization
   S-T segment: neither significantly elevated nor depressed
   T wave: QRS-T angle normal
4. Q-T interval: 0.36 sec.

Impression and Comment

First degree A-V block (borderline)

What appears as first degree A-V block, responds normally, physiologically, with shortening of the P-R interval with exercise in this patient. This electrocardiogram has been unchanged for 20 years and represents this patient's normal electrocardiogram.

Practice
ECG Analysis

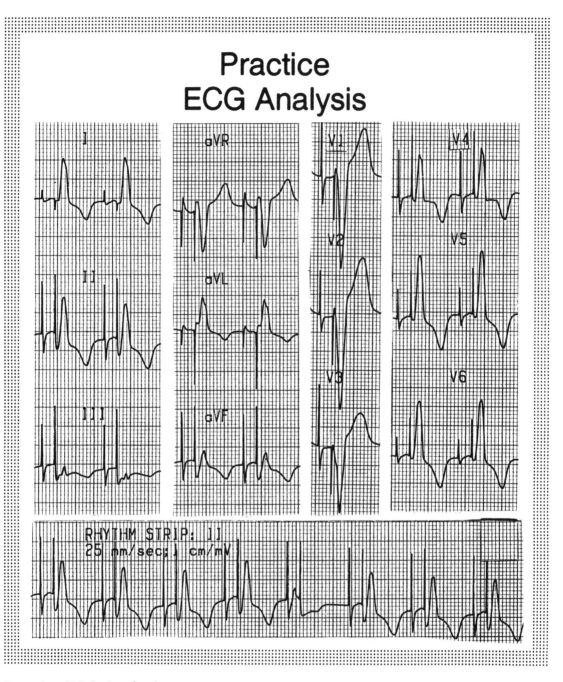

Practice ECG Analysis 18.

The patient is a 73-year-old man with complete (third degree) A-V block and "sick sinus" syndrome.

Analysis:

ECG ANALYSIS 18

1. Rhythm and rate

    Rhythm: artificial sequential atrial and ventricular pacing

    Rate: 88/min.

    P-R interval: 0.14 sec. interval between atrial and ventricular pacemaker impulses

2. QRS complex

    Duration: 0.12 sec.

    Axis: 0°

3. Ventricular repolarization

    S-T segment: depressed in leads I, II, and V_4 to V_6; elevated in leads V_1 to V_3

    T wave: inverted in leads I, II, aVL, and V_4 to V_6; wide QRS-T angle

4. Q-T interval: 0.38 sec.

Impression and Comment

Artificial sequential atrial and ventricular pacing

Ventricular repolarization abnormalities

The artificial atrial and ventricular pacing coordinates the timing of the atrial and ventricular depolarization. This coordination helps maximize cardiac output in this patient with both a "sick sinus" syndrome and third degree A-V block. Because the ventricular pacemaker lead is in the right ventricle, the ventricular pattern in the electrocardiogram is that of a left bundle branch block. The ventricular repolarization abnormalities are predominantly secondary to the depolarization abnormalities.

Practice
ECG Analysis

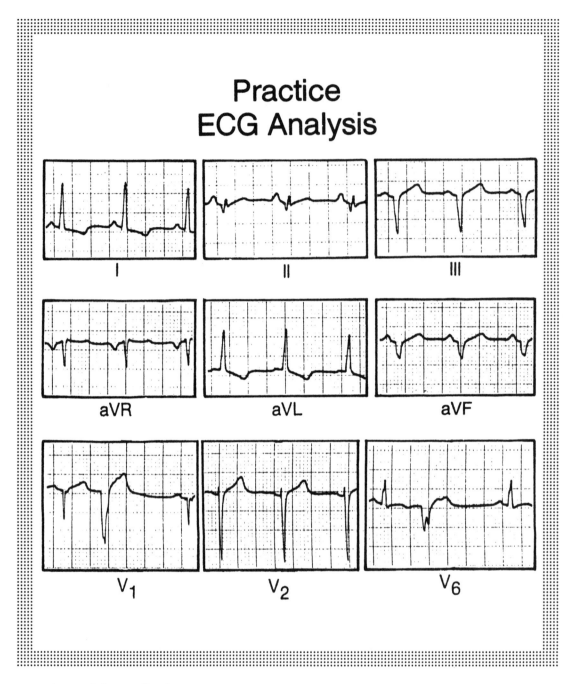

Practice ECG Analysis 19.

The patient is an adult with a history of a heart attack and palpitations.

Analysis:

ECG ANALYSIS 19

1. Rhythm and rate
    Rhythm: sinus
    Rate: 85/min.
    P-R interval: 0.14 sec.
2. QRS complex
    Duration: 0.08 sec.
    Axis: $-25°$
    Significant Q waves in leads II, III, and aVF
    Premature ventricular contractions in leads V_1 and V_6
3. Ventricular repolarization
    S-T segment: depressed in leads I and aVL
    T wave: inverted in leads I, aVL and V_6; wide QRS-T angle
4. Q-T interval: 0.35 sec.

Impression and Comment

Sinus rhythm
Inferior (diaphragmatic) myocardial infarction, old
Left axis deviation
Ventricular repolarization (ST-T) abnormalities
Premature ventricular contractions

There is electrocardiographic evidence of ischemia (ST-T abnormalities) and irritability (premature ventricular contractions) in addition to the old infarction. Careful evaluation is required in view of the already compromised coronary circulation.

Practice
ECG Analysis

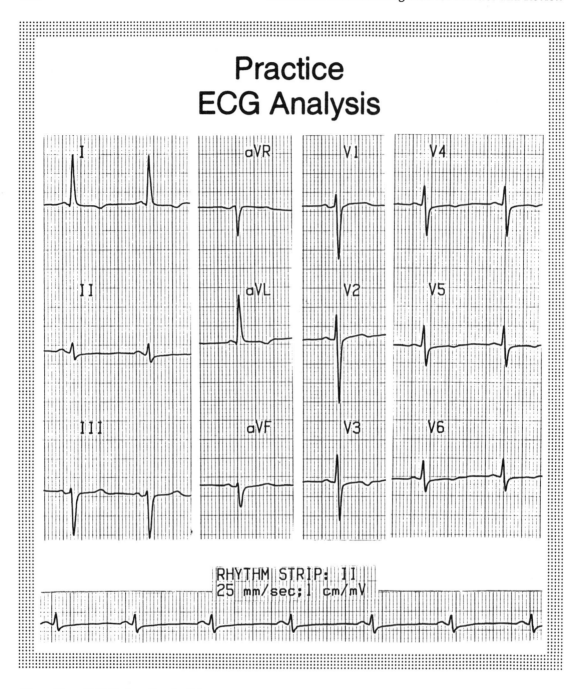

RHYTHM STRIP: II
25 mm/sec; 1 cm/mV

Practice ECG Analysis 20.

The patient is a 78-year-old woman with chest pain on walking, relieved by nitroglycerin.

Analysis:

ECG ANALYSIS 20

1. Rhythm and rate
   Rhythm: sinus
   Rate: 70/min.
   P-R interval: 0.14 sec.
2. QRS complex
   Duration: 0.08 sec.
   Axis: $-30°$
   In the precordial leads, the R wave does not become dominant until lead V_6
3. Ventricular repolarization
   S-T segment: slightly depressed in leads II, V_5, and V_6
   T wave: inverted in leads I, aVL, and V_3 to V_6; QRS-T angle wide
4. Q-T interval: 0.38 sec.

Impression and Comment

Sinus rhythm
Left axis deviation of mean QRS vector
Ventricular repolarization abnormalities, nonspecific
Clockwise rotation
   Evaluation of this patient revealed an ischemic myocardium, secondary to coronary artery disease.

Practice
ECG Analysis

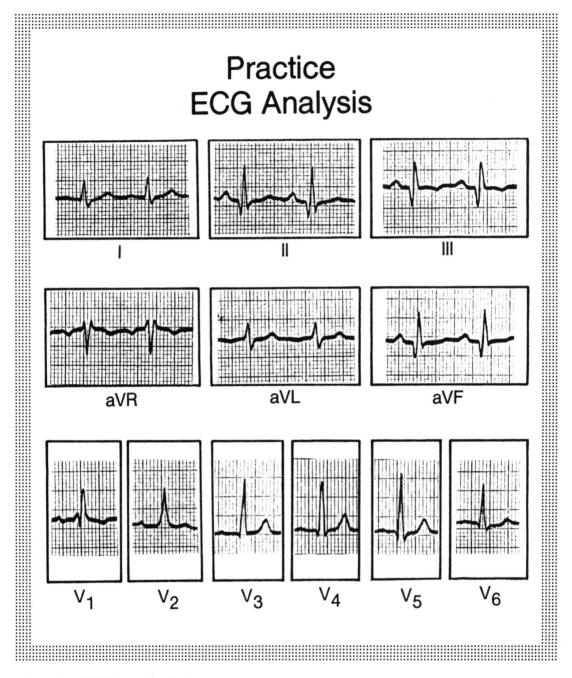

Practice ECG Analysis 21.

The patient is a 65-year-old man with a history of a heart attack 12 years earlier.

Analysis:

ECG ANALYSIS 21

1. Rhythm and rate
   Rhythm: sinus
   Rate: 85/min.
   P-R interval: 0.2 sec.
2. QRS complex
   Duration: 0.12 sec.
   Axis: $+55°$
   QRS complex wide, with an S wave in lead I and an R' in lead V_1
   Significant Q waves in leads II, III and aVF
3. Ventricular repolarization
   S-T segment: neither significantly elevated nor depressed
   T wave: opposite in direction to the terminal deflection of the QRS complex seen best in leads I, II, III, V_1, and V_4 to V_6
4. Q-T interval: 0.36 sec.

Impression and Comment

Sinus rhythm
Inferior (diaphragmatic) myocardial infarction, old
Right bundle branch block (RBBB)
Ventricular repolarization abnormalities (secondary to RBBB)

The significant Q waves in leads II, III and aVF indicate the inferior (diaphragmatic) myocardial infarction. In right bundle branch block the QRS complex is prolonged because of the intraventricular conduction delay. This delay in conduction affects only the *terminal* QRS vector, which is oriented to the *right,* inscribing the S wave in lead I. This terminal QRS vector is also anterior, producing an R' in lead V_1. The *initial* QRS vector is *not* affected by right bundle branch block. The Q waves of myocardial infarction are, therefore, not obscured. The repolarization abnormalities are secondary to the abnormal depolarization in right bundle branch block. The T wave is opposite in direction to the terminal deflection of the QRS complex. This is seen especially well in this electrocardiogram in leads I, II, III, aVR, aVL, V_1, and V_4 to V_6. If this relationship is not present in a patient with right bundle branch block, then additional primary ventricular repolarization abnormalities must be inferred.

Practice
ECG Analysis

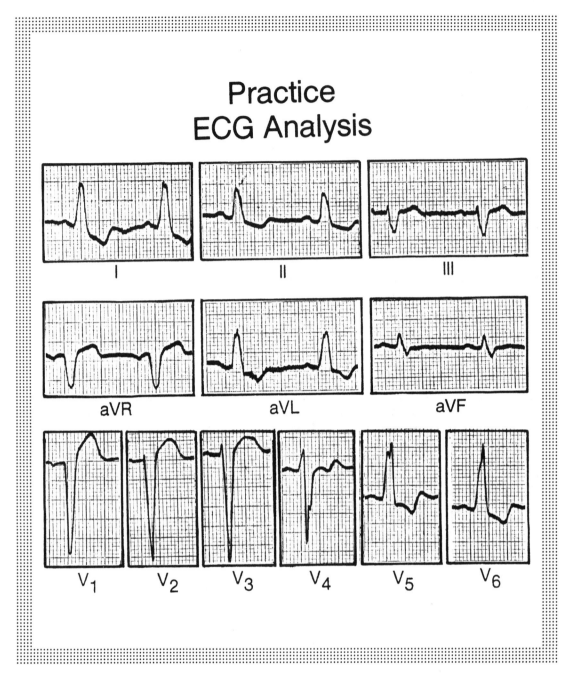

Practice ECG Analysis 22.

The patient is a 70-year-old woman with congestive heart failure.

Analysis:

ECG ANALYSIS 22

1. Rhythm and rate
   Rhythm: sinus
   Rate: 65/min.
   P-R interval: 0.16 sec.
2. QRS complex
   Duration: 0.14 sec.
   Axis: 0°
   QS complex in lead V_1
   Absence of small normal Q waves in leads I, aVL, V_5 and V_6
3. Ventricular repolarization
   S-T segment: depressed in leads I, II, aVL, V_5, and V_6
   T wave: wide QRS-T angle
4. Q-T interval: 0.35 sec.

Impression and Comment

Sinus rhythm
Left bundle branch block (LBBB)
Ventricular repolarization abnormalities
   This patient also had an old inferior (diaphragmatic) myocardial infarction, completely obscured by the development of the left bundle branch block. Left bundle branch block may simulate myocardial infarction electrocardiographically when none has occurred and may mask myocardial infarction in the presence of clear evidence of its occurrence. This patient also had a large left ventricle, which cannot be determined with certainty in the presence of left bundle branch block. Another case of myocardial infarction in the presence of left bundle branch block is presented on pages 308–309.

Practice
ECG Analysis

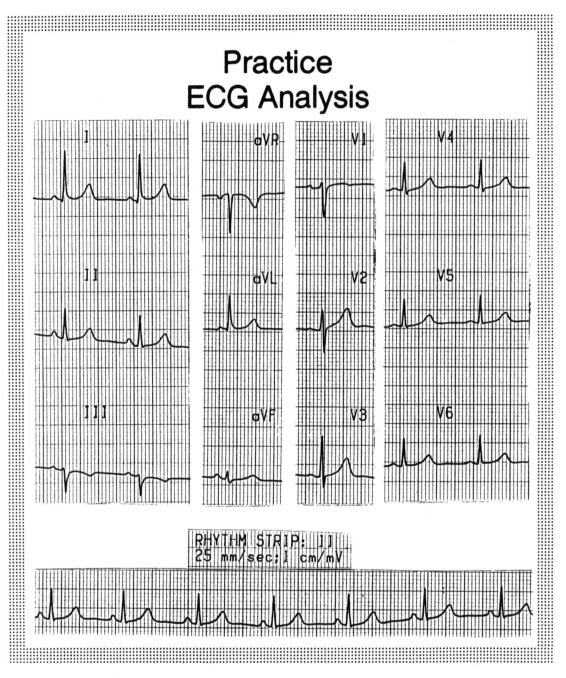

Practice ECG Analysis 23.

The patient is a 48-year-old healthy woman.

Analysis:

ECG ANALYSIS 23

1. Rhythm and rate
    Rhythm: sinus
    Rate: 73/min.
    P-R interval: 0.14 sec.
2. QRS complex
    Duration: 0.08 sec.
    Axis: 0°
3. Ventricular repolarization
    S-T segment: neither significantly elevated nor depressed
    T wave: QRS-T angle normal
4. Q-T interval: 0.36 sec.

Impression and Comment

Normal electrocardiogram

Practice
ECG Analysis

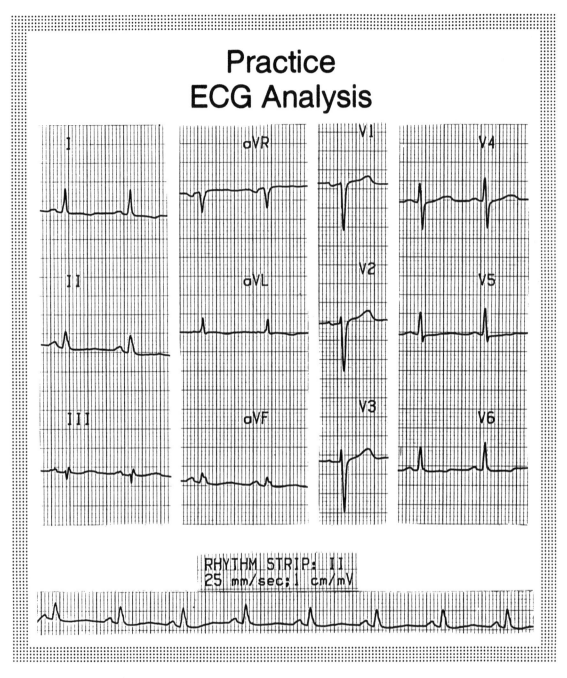

Practice ECG Analysis 24.

The patient is a 47-year-old man with substernal discomfort on effort, relieved by nitroglycerin.

Analysis:

ECG ANALYSIS 24

1. Rhythm and rate
   Rhythm: sinus
   Rate: 85/min.
   P-R interval: 0.16 sec.
2. QRS complex
   Duration: 0.08 sec.
   Axis: $+30°$
3. Ventricular repolarization
   S-T segment: depressed, slightly, in leads I and V_6
   T wave: T waves inverted in leads I, aVL, and V_6; QRS-T angle wide
4. Q-T interval: 0.36 sec.

Impression and Comment

Sinus rhythm

Ventricular repolarization abnormalities; compatible with myocardial ischemia

Full evaluation of this patient did indeed reveal myocardial ischemia due to coronary artery disease.

Practice
ECG Analysis

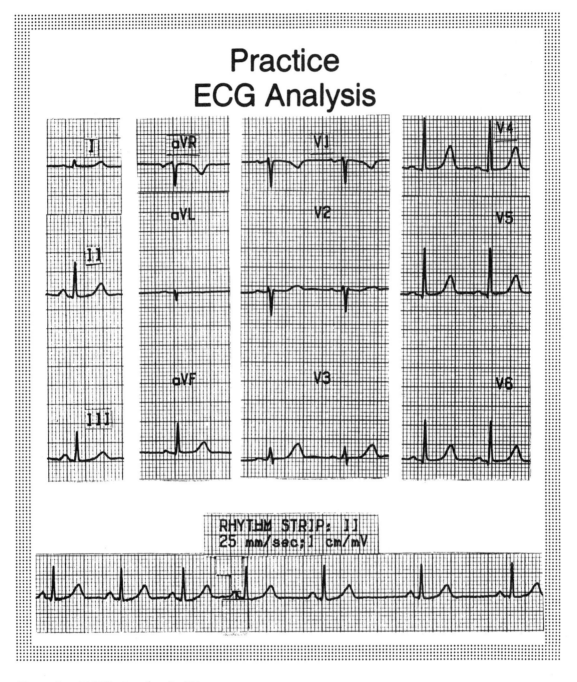

Practice ECG Analysis 25.

The patient is a healthy 18-year-old student.

Analysis:

ECG ANALYSIS 25

1. Rhythm and rate
   Rhythm: sinus
   Rate: 55 to 87/min.
   P-R interval: 0.14 sec.
2. QRS complex
   Duration: 0.06 sec.
   Axis: +75°
3. Ventricular repolarization
   S-T segment: neither significantly elevated nor depressed
   T wave: QRS-T angle normal
4. Q-T interval: 0.32 to 0.4 sec.

Impression and Comment

Sinus arrhythmia

   Note the variation in heart rate, 55 to 87/min., with respective variations in the Q-T interval. Sinus arrhythmia is not uncommon in young people and is not abnormal.

Practice
ECG Analysis

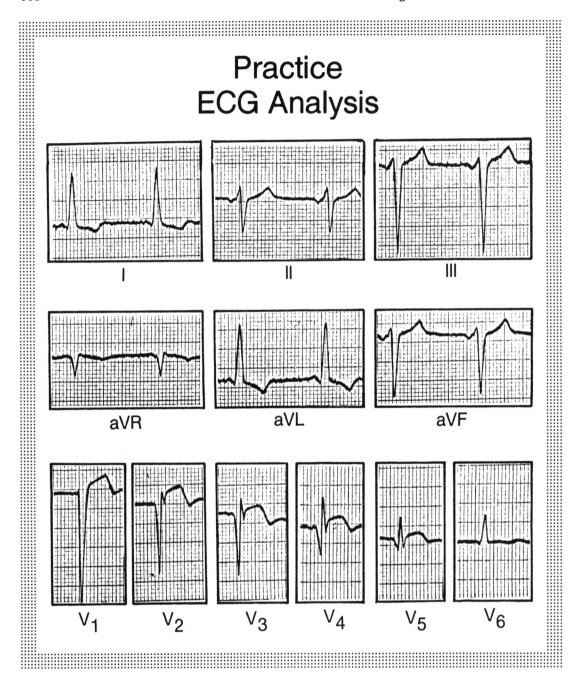

Practice ECG Analysis 26.

The patient is a 78-year-old man who had a heart attack 10 years earlier. He suffers from chronic congestive heart failure.

Analysis:

ECG ANALYSIS 26

1. Rhythm and rate
     Rhythm: A-V junctional
     Rate: 62/min.
     P-R interval: 0.11 sec.
     P waves are positive in lead I and negative in leads II, III, and aVF
2. QRS complex
     Duration: 0.11 sec.
     Axis: $-45°$
     Broad Q waves, best in V_2 to V_5
     The QRS complex in lead V_1 is 30 mm. in size
3. Ventricular repolarization
     S-T segment: elevated and rounded with a "curve of injury" pattern in leads V_1 to V_5
     T wave: inverted in leads I, aVL, and V_4 to V_5 and flat in V_6, where normally they are upright
4. Q-T interval: 0.4 sec.

Impression and Comment

A-V junctional rhythm
Left axis deviation of the mean QRS vector
Ventricular aneurysm
Anterior myocardial infarction, old
Left ventricular hypertrophy
Ventricular repolarization (ST-T) abnormalities
QRS interval prolonged

The P waves are positive in lead I and negative in leads II, III, and aVF, resulting in a left axis deviation of the mean P vector. The negative P waves, together with the short P-R interval, reveal the A-V junctional rhythm. The elevated and rounded S-T segments with a "curve of injury" pattern resembling the evolutionary changes of an acute myocardial infarction represent the ventricular aneurysm. The broad, slurred Q waves, seen especially well in leads V_2 to V_5, reflect the anterior myocardial infarction sustained 10 years earlier. The large size of the QRS complexes, especially lead V_1, of more than 30 mm. signifies left ventricular hypertrophy. The marked ventricular repolarization (ST-T) abnormalities are compatible with the patient's known myocardial ischemia. The prolongation of the QRS interval reveals an intraventricular conduction delay.

Practice
ECG Analysis

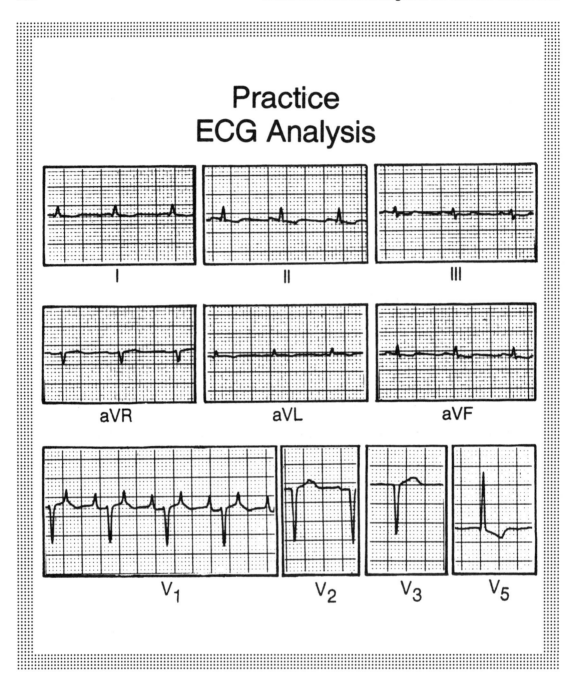

Practice ECG Analysis 27.

The patient is an elderly adult with a history of a heart attack and a heart rhythm disturbance.

Analysis:

ECG ANALYSIS 27

1. Rhythm and rate
   Rhythm: atrial tachycardia (with a 2:1 A-V conduction ratio)
   Rate: atrial, 188/min.; ventricular, 94/min.
   P-R interval: 0.15 sec.
2. QRS complex
   Duration: 0.08 sec.
   Axis: +30°
   Significant Q waves seen best in leads V_2 and V_3
3. Ventricular repolarization
   S-T segment: depressed in leads I, II, and V_5
   T wave: wide QRS-T angle
4. Q-T interval: 0.32 sec.

Impression and Comment

Atrial tachycardia with a 2:1 A-V conduction ratio
Anteroseptal myocardial infarction, old
Ventricular repolarization (ST-T) abnormalities, nonspecific
   The findings on this electrocardiogram emphasize the need to examine the entire electrocardiogram. Without the precordial leads, it would be impossible to come to the above conclusions. Although the frontal plane leads (I, II, III, aVR, aVL, and aVF) reveal an abnormal electrocardiogram with ST-T abnormalities, the precordial leads in the horizontal plane reveal both the arrhythmia and the old myocardial infarction. If the atrial rate were faster (250 to 350 per min.), atrial flutter would be considered.

Practice
ECG Analysis

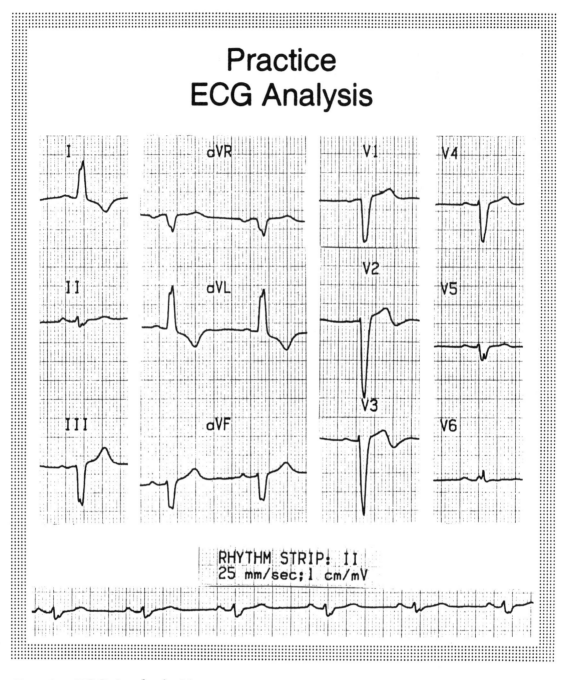

Practice ECG Analysis 28.

The patient is a 79-year-old woman with chest pain for the previous 24 hours.

Analysis:

ECG ANALYSIS 28

1. Rhythm and rate
    Rhythm: sinus
    Rate: 60/min.
    P-R interval: 0.16 sec.
2. QRS complex
    Duration: 0.12 sec.
    axis: $-30°$
    QS complex in lead V_1
3. Ventricular repolarization
    S-T segment: depressed in leads I and aVL and elevated in leads V_1 to V_3
    T wave: inverted in leads I and aVL and biphasic in leads V_2 and V_3
4. Q-T interval: 0.4 sec.

Impression and Comment

Sinus rhythm
Anteroseptal myocardial infarction, acute
Left bundle branch block (LBBB)
Ventricular repolarization abnormalities
Clockwise rotation

The QS complexes are frequently seen in lead V_1 in LBBB and sometimes also in leads V_2 and V_3. These should not be interpreted as findings of anterior or anteroseptal myocardial infarction. In a minority of patients with left bundle branch block, diagnostic Q waves are evident and help in making the diagnosis.[21] Havelda and associates noted that anterior infarction is suggested by a q wave or pathologic Q wave in lead I, a q wave in leads I, V_5, and V_6, or notched S waves in V_3 or V_4.[22]

Repolarization (ST-T) abnormalities will often provide a clue to the presence of myocardial infarction in the presence of left bundle branch block. The acute ST-T changes of myocardial infarction are frequently obvious. The *new* findings of the elevated S-T segment and biphasic T waves in leads V_2 and V_3 are not secondary to the LBBB, but represent the new findings in this patient with anteroseptal myocardial infarction in the presence of LBBB. The myocardial infarction was confirmed by enzyme studies.

Note: Because abnormal depolarization, as occurs in LBBB, is followed by abnormal repolarization, secondarily, it is important to look for new findings, as occurred here, to make the diagnosis of myocardial infarction in the presence of LBBB.

Practice
ECG Analysis

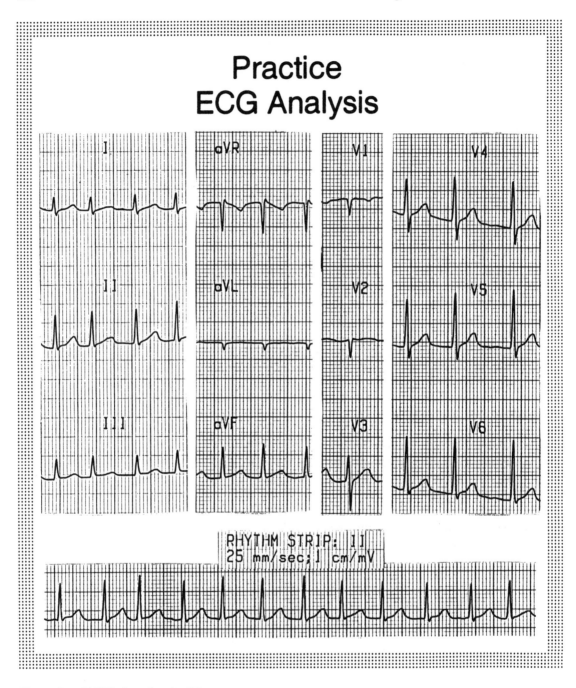

RHYTHM STRIP: II
25 mm/sec; 1 cm/mV

Practice ECG Analysis 29.

The patient is a 55-year-old man with recent onset of shortness of breath and palpitations.

Analysis:

ECG ANALYSIS 29

1. Rhythm and rate
    Rhythm: atrial fibrillation, irregularly irregular
    Rate: 140/min. (average)
    P-R interval: no P waves are present, only fine fibrillatory atrial waves
2. QRS complex
    Duration: 0.08 sec.
    Axis: +65°
3. Ventricular repolarization
    S-T segment: neither significantly elevated nor depressed
    T wave: QRS-T angle within normal limits
4. Q-T interval: 0.28 sec.

Impression and Comment

Atrial fibrillation with rapid ventricular response

The typical irregularly irregular ventricular response that usually accompanies atrial fibrillation is present here. The ventricular rate depends on how many of the 350–600 atrial impulses are conducted to the ventricles. In a patient with recent onset of atrial fibrillation, especially without significant ventricular repolarization abnormalities, evaluation of thyroid function is important since atrial fibrillation may be associated with hyperthyroidism. The aim with therapy is to convert to sinus rhythm. If this cannot be accomplished, the rate must be lowered with medication, e.g., digitalis, to a proper rate for better cardiac output.

Practice
ECG Analysis

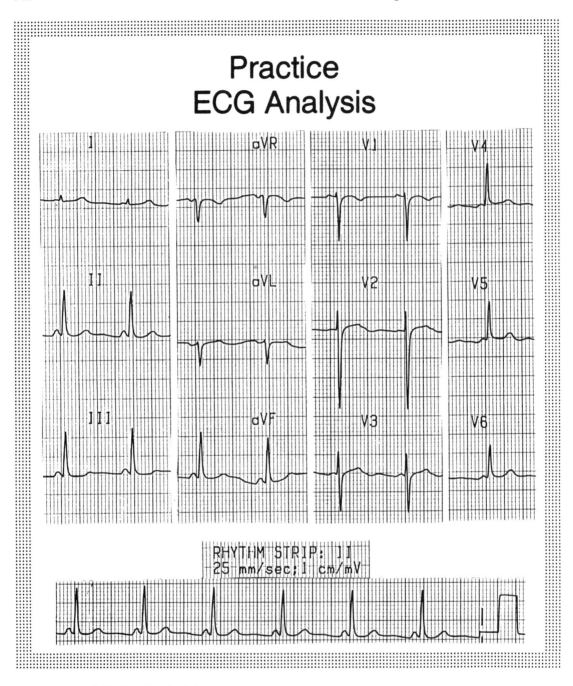

Practice ECG Analysis 30.

The patient is a healthy 26-year-old woman with episodes of palpitations.

Analysis:

ECG ANALYSIS 30

1. Rhythm and rate
    Rhythm: sinus
    Rate: 78/min.
    P-R interval: 0.10 sec.
2. QRS complex
    Duration: 0.08 sec.
    Axis: +85°
3. Ventricular repolarization
    S-T segment: neither significantly elevated nor depressed
    T wave: normal QRS-T angle
4. Q-T interval: 0.34 sec.

Impression and Comment

Sinus rhythm
Short P-R interval (L-G-L) syndrome

The short P-R interval has been associated with various arrhythmias. This was described by Lown, Ganong, and Levine and often called the L-G-L syndrome or the short P-R interval syndrome. Even though no rhythm disturbance is seen in this electrocardiogram, the findings of this syndrome may be a clue to the episodes of palpitations.

Practice
ECG Analysis

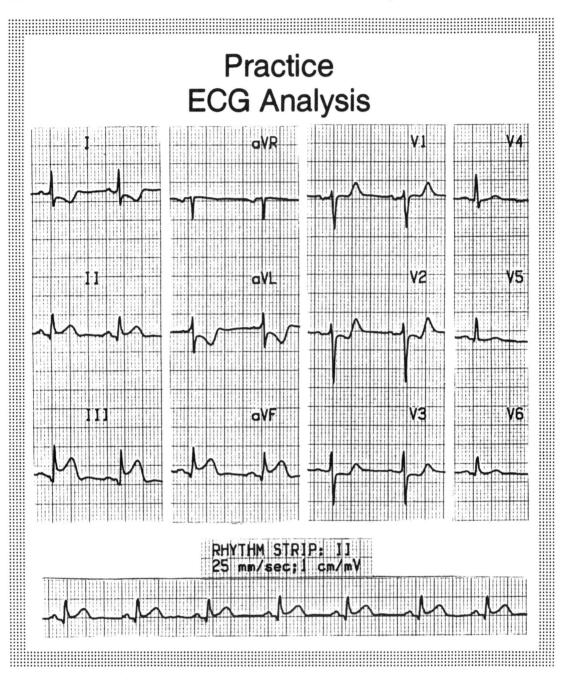

Practice ECG Analysis 31.

The patient is a 40-year-old man who experienced the sudden onset of chest pain several hours earlier.

Analysis:

ECG ANALYSIS 31

1. Rhythm and rate
   Rhythm: sinus
   Rate: 80/min.
   P-R interval: 0.14 sec.
2. QRS complex
   Duration: 0.08 sec.
   Axis: +60°
   Small Q waves in leads II, III, and aVF
3. Ventricular repolarization
   S-T segment: depressed in leads I, aVL, V_2, and V_3 and elevated in leads II, III, and aVF
   T wave: inverted in leads I and aVL, wide QRS-T angle
4. Q-T interval: 0.34 sec.

Impression and Comment

Sinus rhythm

Myocardial infarction, inferior (diaphragmatic), acute

Ventricular repolarization abnormalities, compatible with acute myocardial infarction

Although significant Q waves are not yet evident in leads II, III, and aVF, the elevation of the S-T segment in these leads often signify the acute state (see page 150). Reciprocal changes (see page 369) are seen laterally and anteriorly in leads I, aVL, V_2, and V_3. Additional studies confirmed involvement also of the lateral and posterior walls. Myocardial enzymes were already elevated when this patient arrived. Appropriate therapy during this stage may reverse closure of the affected coronary artery.

Practice
ECG Analysis

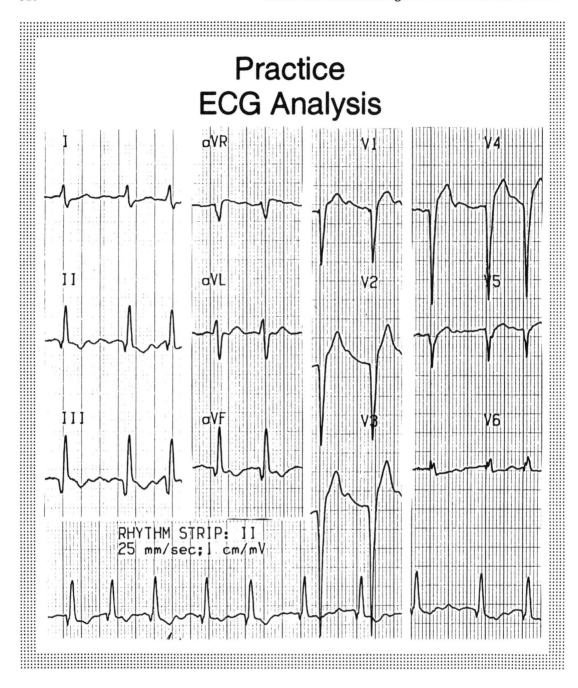

Practice ECG Analysis 32.

The patient is a 75-year-old man with a history of two heart attacks; the first 10 years earlier and the second 6 years earlier. Currently, he is short of breath.

Analysis:

ECG ANALYSIS 32

1. Rhythm and rate
      Rhythm: atrial fibrillation, irregularly irregular
      Rate: 120/min. (average)
      P-R interval: no P waves are present, only fibrillatory atrial waves
2. QRS complex
      Duration: 0.12 sec.
      Axis: $+85°$
      Significant Q waves in leads II, III, aVF, and V_1 to V_5
3. Ventricular repolarization
      S-T segment: depressed in leads I, II, and V_6
      T wave: inverted in leads II, III, and aVF, wide QRS-T angle
4. Q-T interval: 0.3 sec.

Impression and Comment

Atrial fibrillation with rapid ventricular response
Anterior myocardial infarction, old
Inferior (diaphragmatic) myocardial infarction, old
Interventricular conduction disturbance
Ventricular repolarization abnormalities
   Because both myocardial infarctions are old, there is no way of telling which occurred first from this electrocardiogram.

Practice ECG Analysis

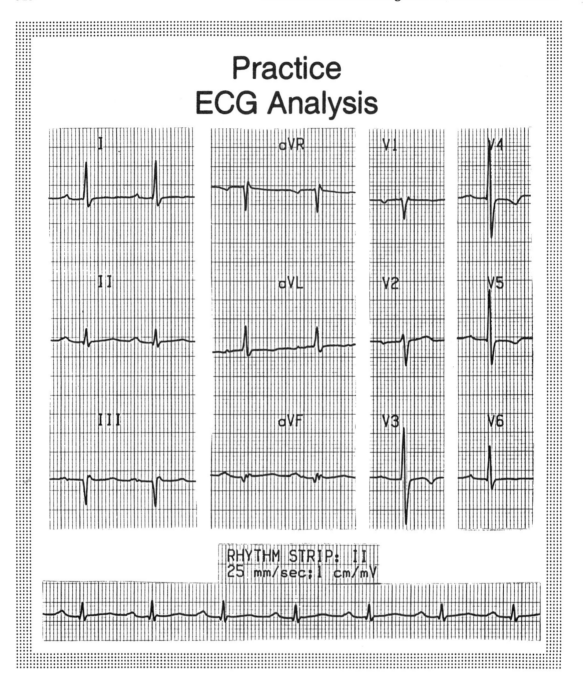

Practice ECG Analysis 33.

The patient is a 66-year-old man with a history of a heart attack 8 years earlier.

Analysis:

ECG ANALYSIS 33

1. Rhythm and rate
   Rhythm: sinus
   Rate: 76/min.
   P-R interval: 0.26 sec.
2. QRS complex
   Duration: 0.08 sec.
   Axis: 0°
   Small Q waves in lead II; significant Q waves in leads III and aVF
3. Ventricular repolarization
   S-T segment: depressed in leads V_4 to V_5
   T wave: wide QRS-T angle
4. Q-T interval: 0.38 sec.

Impression and Comment

First degree A-V block (P-R interval > 0.2 sec.)
Inferior (diaphragmatic) myocardial infarction, old
Ventricular repolarization abnormalities

The first degree A-V block must be carefully watched. If there is progression or advancement to higher degrees of A-V block, artificial pacemaker therapy would be appropriate.

Note: There is an S wave in lead I and a very small R' in lead V_1 with normal QRS duration. Some might call this an incomplete right bundle branch block. This patient was fully evaluated, with no evidence of right bundle branch block. The cause of that very small terminal R wave was found to be positional. It was not present on his other electrocardiograms.

Practice
ECG Analysis

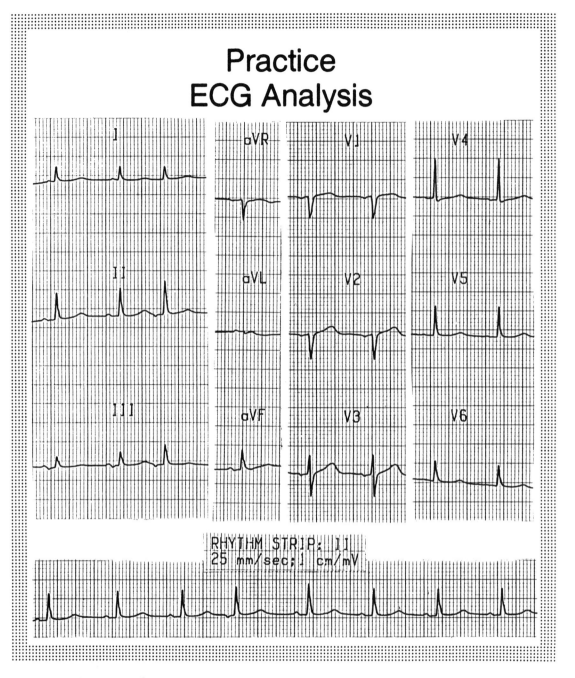

Practice ECG Analysis 34.

The patient is a 77-year-old woman with occasional palpitations.

Analysis:

ECG ANALYSIS 34

1. Rhythm and rate
   Rhythm: sinus (basic rhythm) with premature junctional contractions (PJCs)
   Rate: 86/min. (basic rhythm)
   P-R interval: 0.14 (basic rhythm), 0.10 (PJC)
   In the PJCs the P wave is inverted in leads II and III
2. QRS complex
   Duration: 0.06 sec.
   Axis: $+60°$
3. Ventricular repolarization
   S-T segment: neither significantly elevated nor depressed
   T wave: QRS-T angle normal
4. Q-T interval: 0.34 sec.

Impression and Comment

Sinus rhythm (basic rhythm)
Premature junctional contractions (PJCs)

   The PJCs are seen in simultaneous leads I, II, and III and in the lead II rhythm strip. The mean P vector in these junctional beats is opposite the normal mean P vector, resulting in negative P waves in leads II and III.

Practice
ECG Analysis

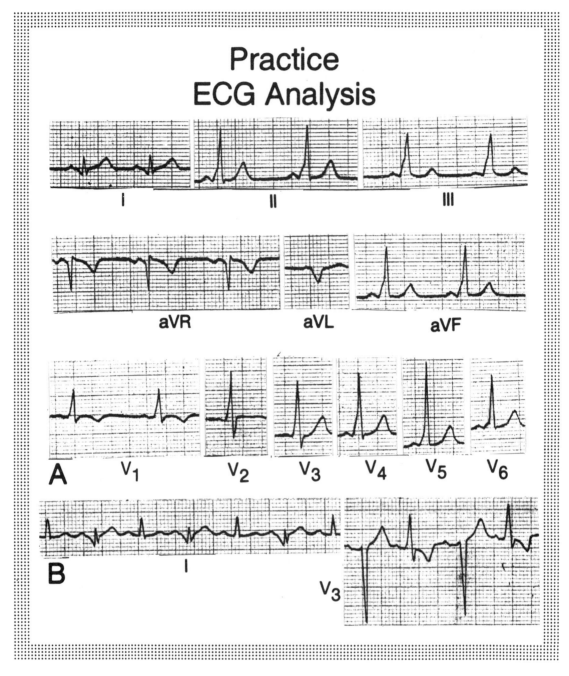

Practice ECG Analysis 35.

The patient is an 18-year-old college student with repeated bouts of very rapid heart rate.

Analysis:

ECG ANALYSIS 35

1. Rhythm and rate

    Rhythm: sinus

    Rate: 70/min. (electrocardiogram A) and 110/min. (rhythm strips B)

    P-R interval: 0.10 sec. (electrocardiogram A) and 0.14 sec. during normal conduction (rhythm strips B)

2. QRS complex

    Duration: 0.12 sec. (electrocardiogram A) and 0.08 sec. during normal conduction (rhythm strip B)

    Axis: +75° (electrocardiogram A)

    The QRS complex has a slurred upstroke (delta wave) in electrocardiogram A and intermittently in rhythm strips B

3. Ventricular repolarization

    S-T segment: neither significantly elevated nor depressed

    T wave: QRS-T angle within normal limits

4. Q-T interval: 0.36 sec.

Impression and Comment

Sinus rhythm

Wolff-Parkinson-White (W-P-W) syndrome

Electrocardiogram A illustrates this patient's W-P-W conduction. Each P wave is followed by a QRS complex starting with the slurred upstroke, known as a delta wave. Rhythm strips B illustrate alternating normal and W-P-W conduction following a period of supraventricular tachycardia. During the tachycardia the heart rate reached 200/min.; even an 18 year old may be quite symptomatic at this persistent rate. Interruption of the accessory pathway solved the problem.

Please note: The delta wave may be negative in some leads (leads I and aVL in electrocardiogram A) and should not be mistaken for the Q wave of myocardial infarction.

Practice
ECG Analysis

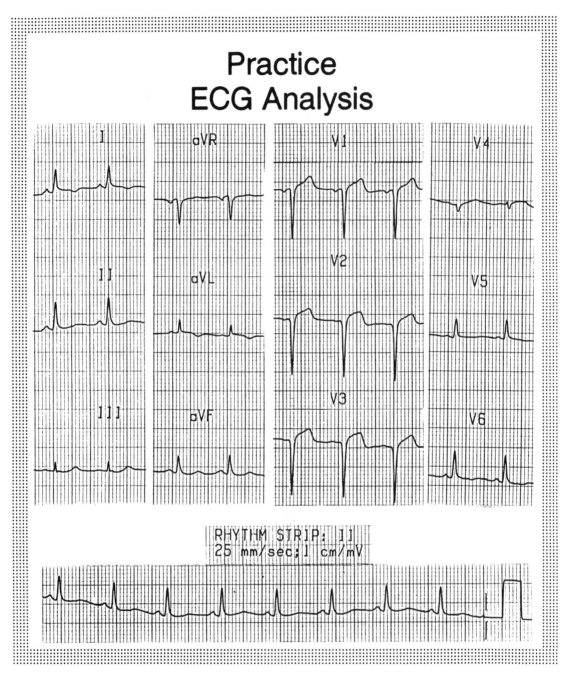

RHYTHM STRIP: II
25 mm/sec; 1 cm/mV

Practice ECG Analysis 36.

The patient is a 48-year-old man who suffered a heart attack 1 week earlier.

Analysis:

ECG ANALYSIS 36

1. Rhythm and rate
    Rhythm: sinus
    Rate: 110/min.
    P-R interval: 0.12 sec.
2. QRS complex
    Duration: 0.08 sec.
    Axis: $+45°$
    QS complexes in leads V_1 to V_3
3. Ventricular repolarization
    S-T segment: elevated, especially leads V_1 to V_3
    T wave: wide QRS-T angle
4. Q-T interval: 0.3 sec.

Impression and Comment

Sinus tachycardia
Anterior myocardial infarction, acute
Ventricular repolarization abnormalities

   Because we do not have an electrocardiogram taken prior to the myocardial infarction, we are unable to determine whether the repolarization abnormalities are the result of the myocardial infarction or were present before. The persistence of these evolutionary changes in ventricular repolarization may also represent a ventricular aneurysm following myocardial infarction.

Practice
ECG Analysis

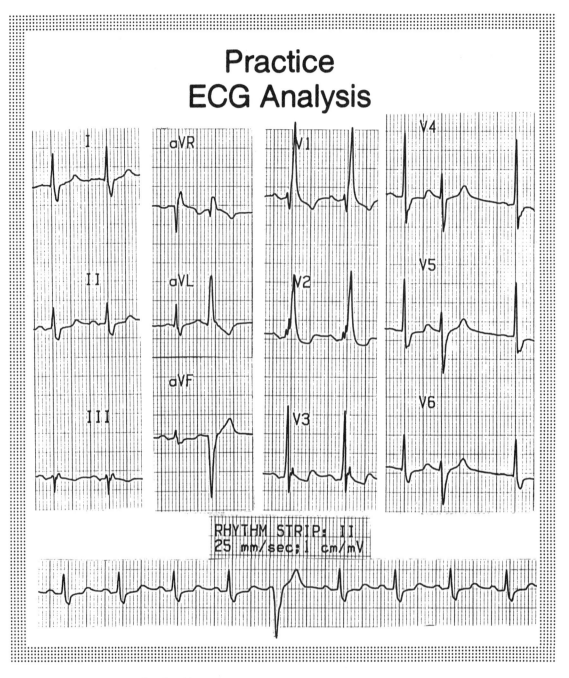

Practice ECG Analysis 42.

The patient is an 80-year-old man with congestive heart failure.

Analysis:

ECG ANALYSIS 37

1. Rhythm and rate
   Rhythm: sinus, with PVCs
   Rate: 98/min.
   P-R interval: 0.16 sec.
2. QRS complex
   Duration: 0.14 sec. in basic rhythm and 0.12 sec. in PVCs
   Axis: $+15°$
   QRS complex in basic rhythm wide with an S wave in lead I and a large terminal R wave in lead V_1
3. Ventricular repolarization
   S-T segment: depressed in leads II and V_2 to V_6
   T wave: opposite in polarity to terminal portion of QRS complex
4. Q-T interval: 0.34 sec.

Impression and Comment

Sinus rhythm
Right bundle branch block (RBBB)
Premature ventricular contractions (PVCs)
Ventricular repolarization abnormalities

Note that the T wave is opposite in polarity to the terminal portion of the QRS complex (leads I, II, III, aVR, aVL, and V_4 to V_6). These changes are secondary to the abnormal ventricular depolarization (RBBB).

Practice
ECG Analysis

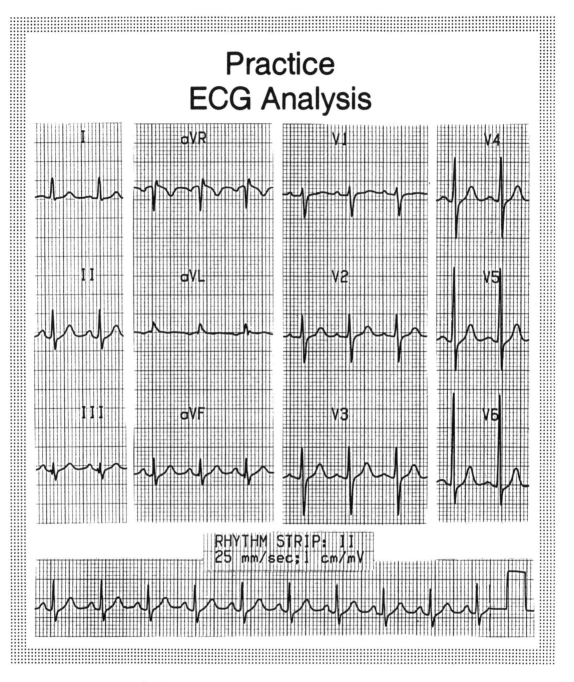

RHYTHM STRIP: II
25 mm/sec; 1 cm/mV

Practice ECG Analysis 38.

The patient is a healthy 20-year-old man following physical exertion.

Analysis:

ECG ANALYSIS 38

1. Rhythm and rate
    Rhythm: sinus
    Rate: 115/min.
    P-R interval: 0.14 sec.
2. QRS complex
    Duration: 0.08 sec.
    Axis: +30°
3. Ventricular repolarization
    S-T segment: neither significantly elevated nor depressed
    T wave: QRS-T angle normal
4. Q-T interval: 0.32 sec.

Impression and Comment

Sinus tachycardia
    This electrocardiogram is normal in a 20-year-old man following physical exertion.

Practice
ECG Analysis

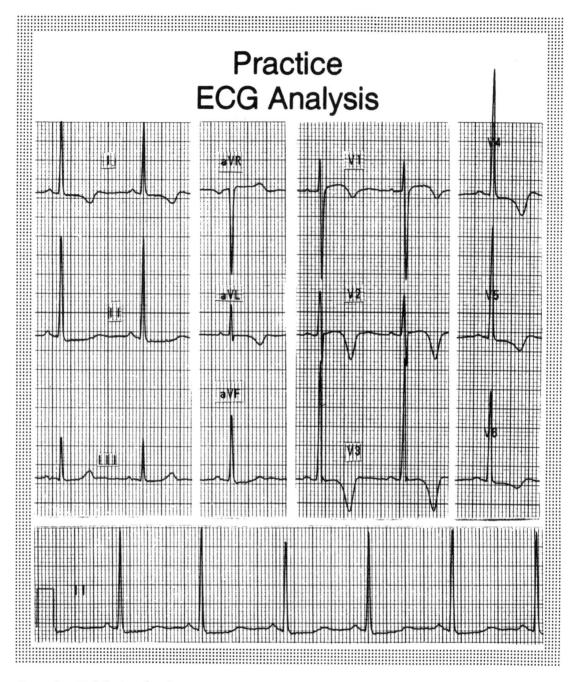

Practice ECG Analysis 39.

The patient is a 55-year-old woman with a history of hypertension, angina pectoris on effort, and onset of chest pain, unrelieved by nitroglycerin, 3 days earlier.

Analysis:

ECG ANALYSIS 39

1. Rhythm and rate
     Rhythm: sinus
     Rate: 65/min.
     P-R interval: 0.16 sec.
2. QRS complex
     Duration: 0.08 sec.
     Axis: $+45°$
     $S_{v1} + R_{v5} = 53$ mm.
3. Ventricular repolarization
     S-T segment: depressed in lead II; elevated with appearance of curve of injury in leads V_1 and V_2
     T wave: deeply inverted in leads V_2 to V_4; wide QRS-T angle
4. Q-T interval: 0.4 sec.

Impression and Comment

Sinus rhythm

Myocardial infarction, anterior (with no Q waves), acute

Left ventricular hypertrophy

Ventricular repolarization abnormalities

This patient had clinical and enzyme abnormalities compatible with myocardial infarction. This is reflected electrocardiographically in the curve of injury in leads V_1 and V_2 and the deeply inverted T waves in leads V_2 to V_4. Left ventricular hypertrophy is generally accompanied by secondary repolarization abnormalities; the repolarization abnormalities resulting from the myocardial infarction are additive to those secondary abnormalities.

Practice
ECG Analysis

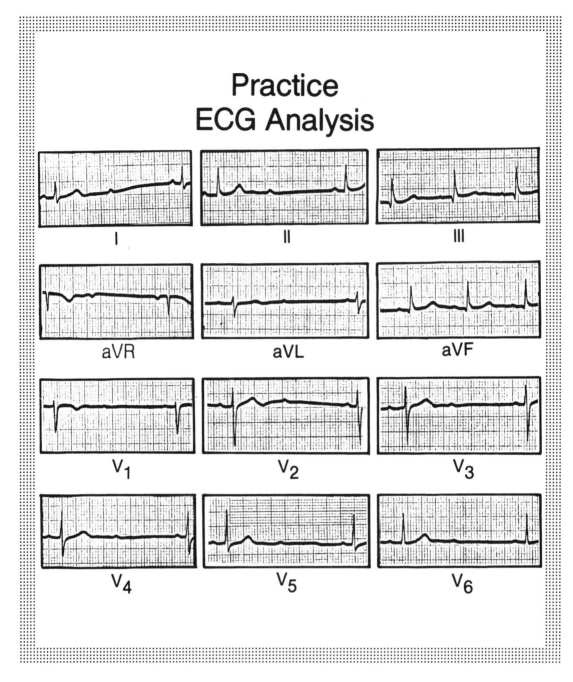

Practice ECG Analysis 40.

The patient is a 68-year-old woman with a complaint of intermittent dizziness.

Analysis:

ECG ANALYSIS 40

1. Rhythm and rate
    Rhythm: second degree A-V block with 2:1 A-V conduction (except leads III and aVF, where there is 1:1 conduction)
    Rate: atrial, 68/min.; ventricular, 34/min.
    Varying P-R intervals, 0.16 to 0.20 sec. (conducted beats)
2. QRS complex
    Duration: 0.08 sec.
    Axis: +75°
3. Ventricular repolarization
    S-T segment: normal, neither significantly elevated nor depressed
    T wave: QRS-T angle normal
4. Q-T interval: 0.4 sec.

Impression and Comment

Second degree (2:1) A-V block

   The patient had intermittent second degree A-V block with a ventricular rate of 34 per min., which was not sufficient to sustain her comfortably. The conducted beats reveal considerable variation in P-R intervals, providing a clue as to the problem even when her A-V conduction is 1:1. Artificial pacemaker therapy gave her complete relief of symptoms.

Practice
ECG Analysis

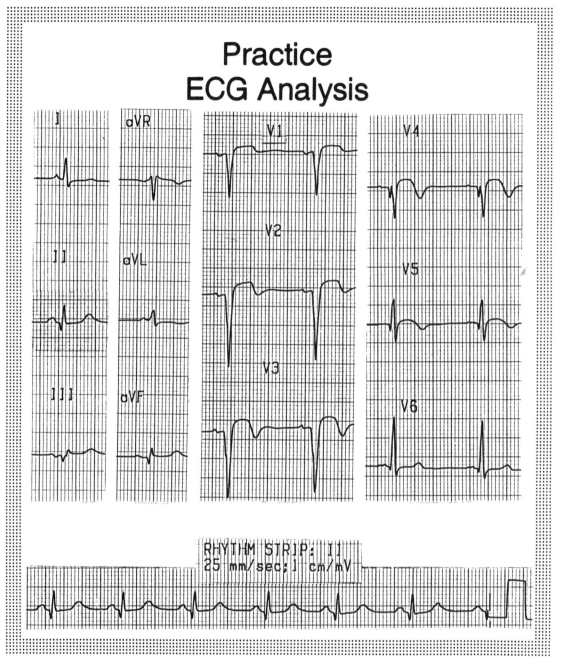

Practice ECG Analysis 41.

The patient is a 49-year-old man with history of a heart attack 5 years earlier and recent onset of severe chest pain.

Analysis:

ECG ANALYSIS 41

1. Rhythm and rate
    Rhythm: sinus
    Rate: 70/min.
    P-R interval: 0.12 sec.
2. QRS complex
    Duration: 0.1 sec.
    Axis: $+15°$
    Significant Q waves in leads II, III, aVF, and V_1 to V_4
3. Ventricular repolarization
    S-T segment: monophasic curves of injury in leads V_1 to V_5, appear to be evolving
    T wave: inverted in leads V_2 to V_5; biphasic in lead V_1
4. Q-T interval: 0.36 sec.

Impression and Comment

Sinus rhythm
Inferior (diaphragmatic) myocardial infarction, old
Anterior myocardial infarction, recent
Ventricular repolarization abnormalities compatible with myocardial infarction, recent

   If we did not have the history of recent chest pain, enzyme studies, and other electrocardiograms for comparison, the electrocardiographic patterns in leads V_1 to V_5 could represent a ventricular aneurysm following an old myocardial infarction.

Practice
ECG Analysis

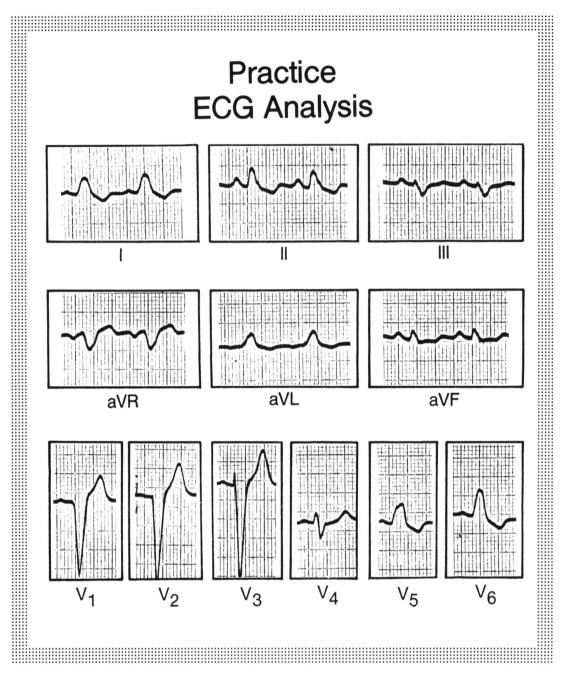

Practice ECG Analysis 42.

The patient is an 80-year-old man with congestive heart failure.

Analysis:

ECG ANALYSIS 42

1. Rhythm and rate
    Rhythm: sinus
    Rate: 90/min.
    P-R interval: 0.18 sec.
2. QRS complex
    Duration: 0.16 sec.
    Axis: $+15°$
    QS complexes in leads V_1 and V_2
    Absence of the small normal Q waves in leads I, aVL, V_5, and V_6
3. Ventricular repolarization
    S-T segment: depressed in leads I, II, aVF, V_5, and V_6
    T wave: inverted in leads I, II, V_5, and V_6, wide QRS-T angle
4. Q-T interval: 0.35 sec.

Impression and Comment

Sinus rhythm
Left bundle branch block
Ventricular repolarization abnormalities
    Review the criteria for left bundle branch block. All are present here.
    1. The QRS interval is 0.16 sec.
    2. QS complexes in leads V_1 and V_2.
    3. Absence of small normal Q waves in leads I, aVL, V_5, and V_6.
    4. Marked ventricular repolarization abnormalities.

The QS complexes in leads V_1 and V_2 are the result of the left bundle branch and should *not* be interpreted as anterior or anteroseptal myocardial infarction. When ventricular depolarization is abnormal, as occurs in left bundle branch block, ventricular repolarization is also abnormal, as seen in this electrocardiogram.

Practice
ECG Analysis

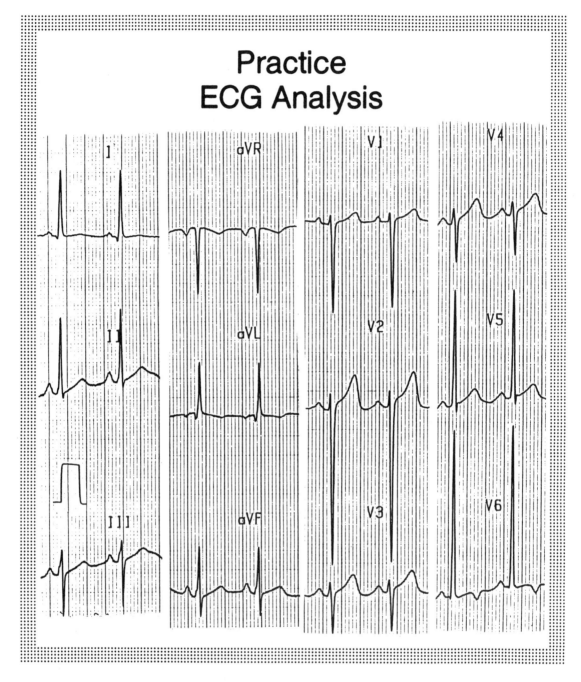

Practice ECG Analysis 43.

The patient is a 42-year-old woman with a history of hypertension.

Analysis:

ECG ANALYSIS 43

1. Rhythm and rate
     Rhythm: sinus
     Rate: 92/min.
     P-R interval: 0.14 sec.
2. QRS complex
     Duration: 0.08 sec.
     Axis: +15°
     $S_{v2} + R_{v6} = 75$ mm.
3. Ventricular repolarization
     S-T segment: not significantly elevated nor depressed
     T wave: low in lead I, inverted in leads aVL and V_6, wide QRS-T angle
4. Q-T interval: 0.36 sec.

Impression and Comment

Sinus rhythm
Left ventricular hypertrophy
Ventricular repolarization abnormalities

   The two major electrocardiographic criteria for left ventricular hypertrophy are met here: increased magnitude of the QRS complexes and ventricular repolarization abnormalities.

Practice
ECG Analysis

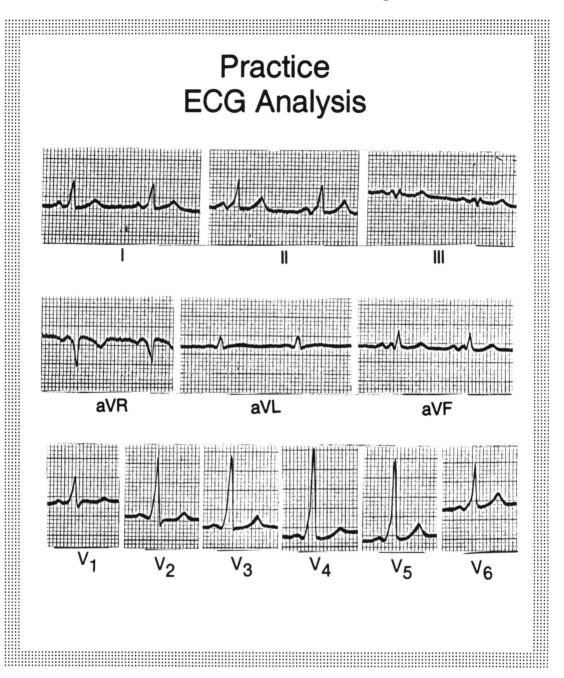

Practice ECG Analysis 44.

The patient is a 65-year-old man with a lifelong history of episodic palpitations.

Analysis:

ECG ANALYSIS 44

1. Rhythm and rate
    Rhythm: sinus
    Rate: 70/min.
    P-R interval: 0.10 sec.
2. QRS complex
    Duration: 0.14 sec.
    Axis: $+30°$
    The QRS complex has a slurred upstroke (delta wave)
3. Ventricular repolarization
    S-T segment: neither significantly elevated nor depressed
    T wave: normal QRS-T angle
4. Q-T interval: 0.4 sec.

Impression and Comment

Sinus rhythm

Wolff-Parkinson-White (W-P-W) syndrome

This syndrome, caused by a bypass tract such as the Kent bundle, is often associated with supraventricular tachycardias. This patient had multiple episodes of rapid heart action throughout his life but was not troubled with chest pain until he entered his sixties. At this age a sudden rate of 180/min. provoked angina pectoris. Interruption of the accessory pathway solved the problem.

In some patients with this syndrome, the electrocardiographic recognition may be quite elusive, with the delta wave appearing only after an episode of tachycardia. The W-P-W syndrome must be suspected in a patient with a history of multiple episodes of tachycardia.

Practice
ECG Analysis

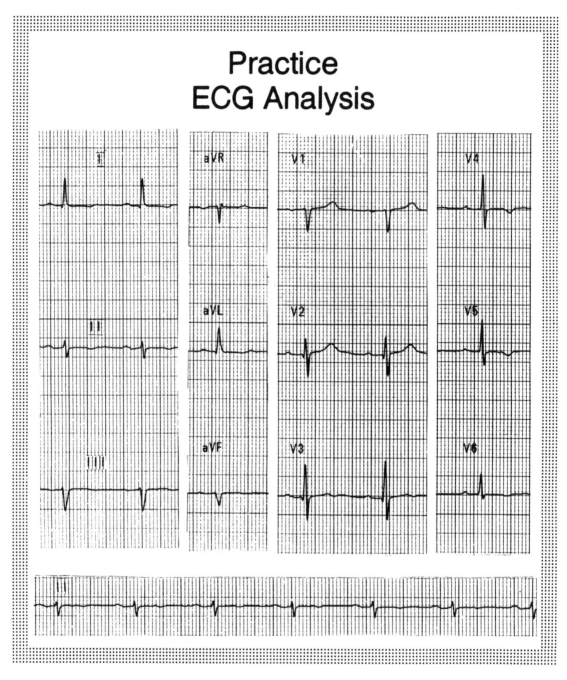

Practice ECG Analysis 45.

The patient is a 59-year-old man with a history of angina pectoris on effort. He suffered a myocardial infarction 10 years earlier.

Analysis:

ECG ANALYSIS 45

1. Rhythm and rate
   Rhythm: sinus
   Rate: 70/min.
   P-R interval: 0.20 sec.
2. QRS complex
   Duration: 0.08 sec.
   Axis: $-30°$
   QS complex in lead V_1 and small pretransitional Q wave in lead V_2
3. Ventricular repolarization
   S-T segment: neither significantly elevated nor depressed
   T wave: inverted in leads I and V_4 to V_6, QRS-T angle wide
4. Q-T interval: 0.36 sec.

Impression and Comment

Sinus rhythm
Left axis deviation of the mean QRS vector
Anteroseptal myocardial infarction, old
Ventricular repolarization abnormalities

The only vestige of the documented anteroseptal myocardial infarction is the QS complex in lead V_1 and the small pretransitional Q wave in lead V_2.

Practice
ECG Analysis

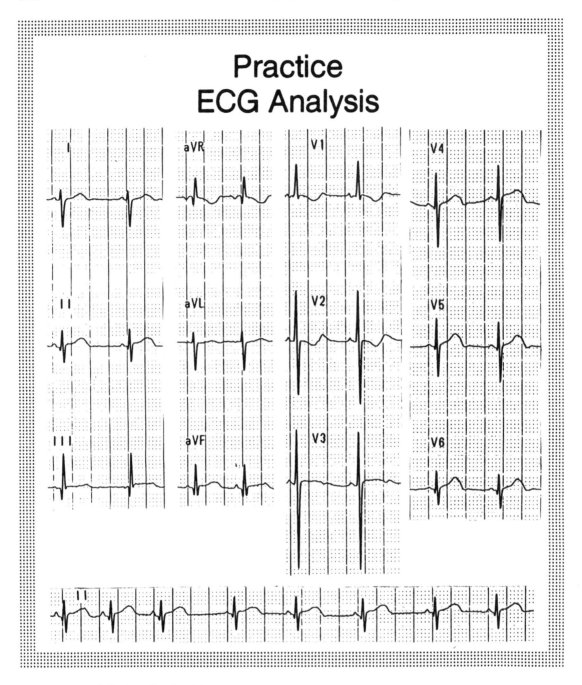

Practice ECG Analysis 46.

The patient is a normal healthy male at 3 days of age.

Analysis:

ECG ANALYSIS 46

1. Rhythm and rate

    Rhythm: sinus arrhythmia

    Rate: 90/min. (average)

    P-R interval: 0.12 sec.

2. QRS complex

    Duration: 0.08 sec.

    Axis: +150°

3. Ventricular repolarization

    S-T segment: slight variations, within normal limits

    T wave: upright in leads I, II, and V_4 to V_6; negative in lead V_1 (see comment below)

4. Q-T interval: 0.32 sec.

Impression and Comment

Sinus arrhythmia

Normal electrocardiogram in a three-day-old infant

Although this is not a course in pediatric electrocardiography, it is important to appreciate the normal newborn electrocardiogram as well as the changes occurring in early life (see page 360).

Some of the principal electrocardiographic findings in the first week of life include:[23]

1. Right axis deviation (to 180°) of the mean QRS vector

2. R wave prominent in lead V_1 (see page 360) with an R/S ratio >1

3. Reversal of R/S progression in the precordial leads

4. The T wave in lead V_1 becomes negative by the age of three days; if the T wave in lead V_1 remains upright by the third day, right ventricular hypertrophy should be suspected.

Practice
ECG Analysis

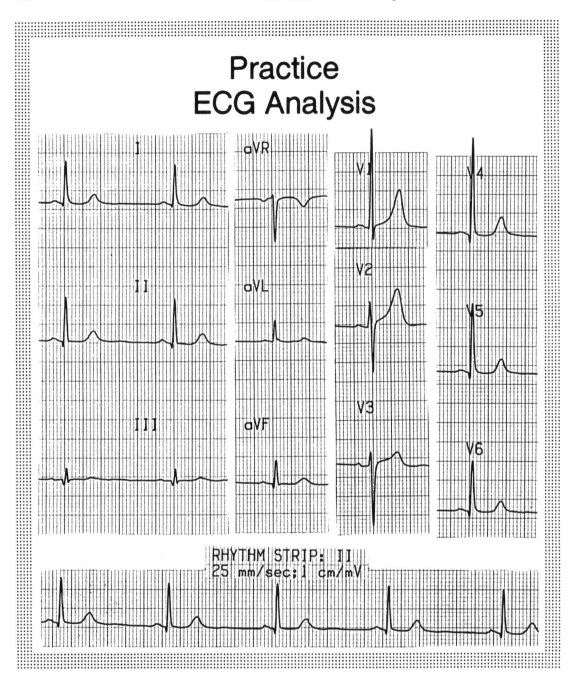

Practice ECG Analysis 47.

The patient is a 56-year-old healthy, athletic man.

Analysis:

ECG ANALYSIS 47

1. Rhythm and rate
   Rhythm: sinus
   Rate: 50/min.
   P-R interval: 0.14 sec.
2. QRS complex
   Duration: 0.08 sec.
   Axis: +45°
3. Ventricular repolarization
   S-T segment: neither significantly elevated nor depressed
   T wave: QRS-T angle normal
4. Q-T interval: 0.42 sec.

Impression and Comment

Sinus bradycardia

This is a normal electrocardiogram in this healthy, athletic 56-year-old man. Note that the Q-T interval of 0.42 sec. is not prolonged with a heart rate of 50/min.

Practice
ECG Analysis

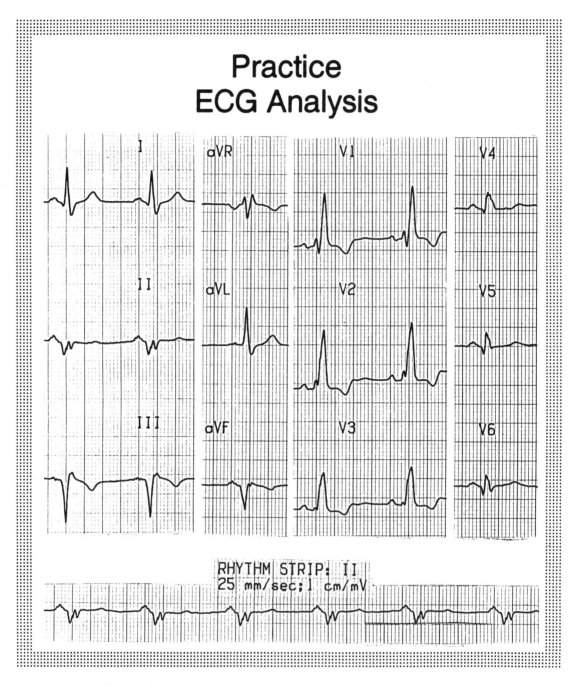

Practice ECG Analysis 48.

The patient is a 56-year-old man with a history of a heart attack 8 years earlier.

Analysis:

ECG ANALYSIS 48

1. Rhythm and rate
   Rhythm: sinus
   Rate: 65/min.
   P-R interval: 0.16 sec.
2. QRS complex
   Duration: 0.14 sec.
   Axis: $-60°$ based on transitional lead aVR
   QRS complex wide, with an S wave in lead I and an R' in lead V_1
   Significant Q waves in leads II, III, aVF, V_5 and V_6
3. Ventricular repolarization
   S-T segment: depressed in leads V_2 and V_3
   T wave: opposite in direction to the terminal deflection of the QRS complex, seen best in leads I, II, III, V_3, and V_5 and V_6
4. Q-T interval: 0.4 sec.

Impression and Comment

Sinus rhythm
Inferior (diaphragmatic) lateral myocardial infarction, old
Right bundle branch block (RBBB)
Left axis deviation (LAD) of the mean QRS vector
Ventricular repolarization abnormalities
   Eight years earlier, the inferolateral myocardial infarction, right bundle branch block, and left axis deviation occurred simultaneously. It is presumed that bifascicular block (RBBB + LAD) is present even though not all the criteria are present.

Practice
ECG Analysis

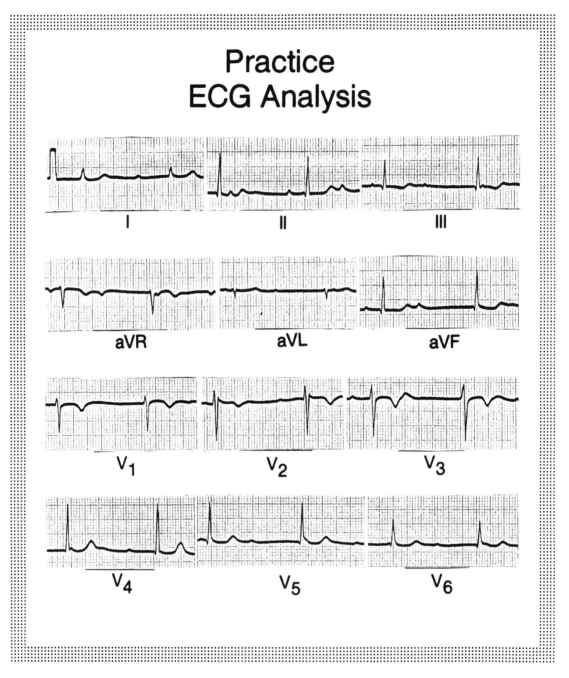

Practice ECG Analysis 49.

The patient is an asymptomatic high school student.

Analysis:

ECG ANALYSIS 49

1. Rhythm and rate

   Rhythm: third degree (complete) A-V block

   Rate: 70/min. (atrial); 45/min. (ventricular)

   P-R interval: because no relationship exists between the atria and the ventricles there is no measurable P-R interval

2. QRS complex

   Duration: 0.08 sec.

   Axis: +75°

3. Ventricular repolarization

   S-T segment: neither significantly elevated nor depressed

   T wave: QRS-T angle normal

4. Q-T interval: 0.44 sec.

Impression and Comment

Third degree (complete) A-V block, congenital

   The patient is an asymptomatic 18-year-old student with congenital third degree (complete) A-V block. There is no relationship between the atria and the ventricles. The atria are under the control of the S-A node and the ventricles are under the control of the A-V junction. The Q-T interval of 0.44 sec. is normal at a ventricular rate of 45/min.

Practice
ECG Analysis

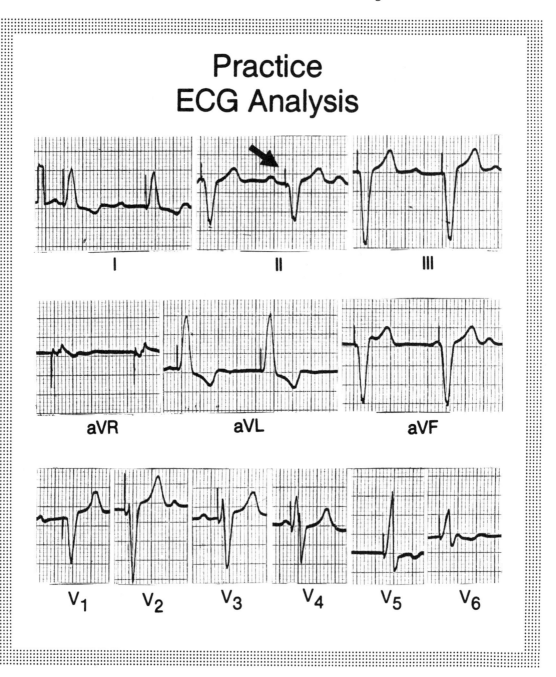

Practice ECG Analysis 50.

The patient is a 74-year-old man who suddenly developed a very low ventricular rate.

Analysis:

ECG ANALYSIS 50

1. Rhythm and rate
   Rhythm: ventricular pacing
   Rate: 82/min. (atrial); 65/min. (ventricular)
   P-R interval: there is no relationship between the P waves and the QRS complexes, hence no measurable P-R interval
2. QRS complex
   Duration: 0.14 sec.
   Axis: $-60°$
3. Ventricular repolarization
   S-T segment: depressed in leads I, aVL, and V_6; elevated in leads II, III, and aVF
   T wave: wide QRS-T angle
4. Q-T interval: 0.4 sec.

Impression and Comment

Third degree (complete) A-V block
Artificial ventricular pacing
LBBB pattern
Ventricular repolarization abnormalities

This patient, whose electrocardiogram had been normal, developed third degree (complete) A-V block with a low ventricular rate, requiring artificial pacemaker therapy. Because the catheter was placed in the right ventricle, the electrocardiogram reveals a left bundle branch block pattern. The repolarization abnormalities are secondary to the abnormal depolarization. Subsequently, this patient was treated with sequential atrial and ventricular pacing, which resulted in atrial and ventricular coordination.

Notes and References

NOTES

From Page 67: Ladder Diagram (Laddergram)

The ladder diagram or laddergram is a useful aid in the study of normal and abnormal rhythms of the heart. It is a method of visually displaying the timing of events. The ladder consists of at least three levels. A represents atrial depolarization, the P wave. V represents ventricular depolarization, the QRS complex. A-V represents atrioventricular conduction across the atrioventricular junction. The S-A node is at the top of the A level. A ladder diagram of normal sinus rhythm and the three steps in its construction is presented.

Step 1. The onset of atrial depolarization, the P wave, is indicated in the A level.

Step 2. The onset of ventricular depolarization, the QRS complex, is indicated in the V level.

Step 3. The line in the A-V level, connecting the atria with the ventricles indicates conduction through the A-V junction. The delay in A-V conduction is shown by the slope of the line in this level.

Note that the A and V level lines have a slight slope in the direction of the passage of the impulse. Often, however, depolarization of the atria and ventricles is indicated by straight vertical lines in the A and V levels, connected by a sloping line through the A-V level. The dot (●), representing the site of impulse formation, and the arrow (▼), showing the direction of conduction, have been added for graphic completeness but are not strictly needed because the timing of events with the sloping line through the A-V level is sufficient to indicate the direction of conduction.

From Page 67 (continued)

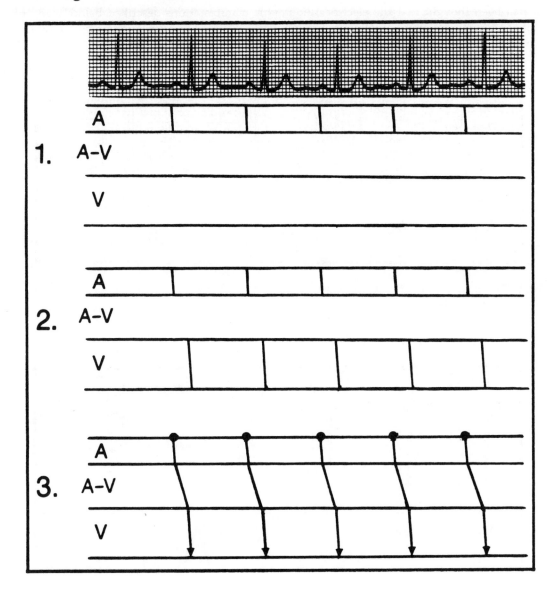

From Page 77: *Clockwise and Counterclockwise Rotation*[24,25]

It had been thought that the electrocardiographic manifestations described below were the result of anatomic rotation; actually, very little rotation occurs. The terms *clockwise* and *counterclockwise rotation* are still in use, but should be used in an electrical sense only.

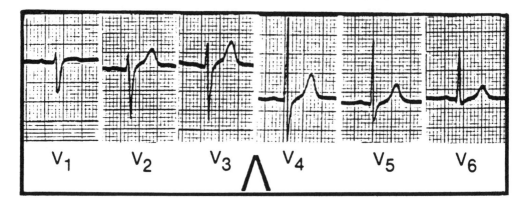

Normal. The transition from predominantly S waves to predominantly R waves occurs in lead V_3 or V_4 or between them. In this electrocardiogram the transition occurs between leads V_3 and V_4.

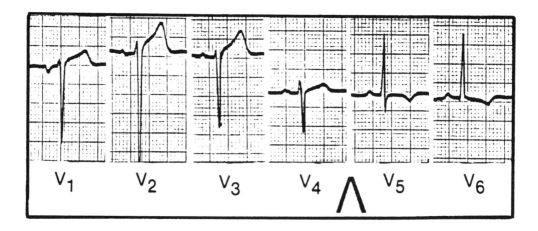

Clockwise rotation. The transition occurs beyond lead V_4. In this electrocardiogram the transition occurs between leads V_4 and V_5. Schamroth refers to clockwise rotation when rS or RS patterns are present in all or most of the precordial leads.

From Page 77 (continued)

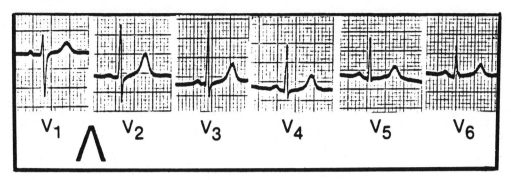

Counterclockwise rotation. The transition occurs before lead V_3. In this electrocardiogram the transition occurs between leads V_1 and V_2.

Other terms, less commonly used today, described the electrical position of the heart. These include the terms horizontal, vertical, semihorizontal, semivertical, and intermediate. It is much more common to state that the mean electrical axes are 0°, 45°, or 90° than to refer to those hearts as horizontal, intermediate, or vertical, respectively.

From Page 97

TABLE 2-1. Right Ventricular Hypertrophy

Once the basic concepts of the vectorial forces of right ventricular and right and left atrial enlargement are understood, the criteria are easily learned. The emphasis in this course has always been on the concept rather than on the "criteria." Do not be a slave to figures; they frequently change in the face of evolving information. The following values are general, especially for infants and children in whom the changes progress rapidly during the first few years.

A. Right Axis Deviation (RAD)
   Evaluate carefully since right axis deviation is normal in the very young.

B. Magnitude of the Mean QRS Vector
   Frontal Plane Leads: I, II, III, aVR, aVL, and aVF.
   Incomplete right bundle branch block (RBBB) pattern. RBBB is discussed and illustrated in Chapter 5.

   $S_I + R_{III}$ and/or $S_{aVL} + R_{aVF} \geq 35$ mm. (principally in children)

   RaVR or R'aVR $\geq$ **6mm.**
   RaVR > QaVR
   The R in lead aVR becomes taller with increased magnitude of the mean QRS vector, especially as the vector becomes more rightward (toward + aVR).

   Horizontal Plane Leads: V_1 to V_6.
   Algebraic sum of R and S waves in lead V_1 more than 15 mm. in height,
   At birth a tall R wave in lead V_1 may still be normal. An R wave in lead V_1 greater than 15 mm., however, may represent an abnormally enlarged right ventricle even in the newborn.

R-S, from Nadas and Fyler,[26] gives the algebraic sum of the R and S waves in lead V_1 from birth to 13 years. For example, if at birth the algebraic sum of the R and S waves is 25 mm., which is well outside the normal range, right ventricular hypertrophy is strongly suggested.

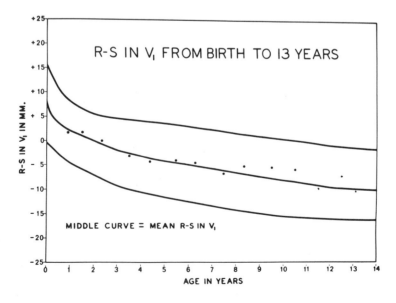

The algebraic sum of R and S waves in lead V_1 from birth to 13 years. The progression of the mean QRS vector in the horizontal plane, from anterior to posterior is reflected in the R-S ratio in lead V_1. (From Nadas, A. S., and Fyler, D. C.: Pediatric Cardiology, 3rd Ed. Philadelphia, W. B. Saunders, 1972).

From Page 97 (continued)

Note: In an adult, if the R wave is the main ventricular deflection in lead V_1, regardless of size, the possibility of right ventricular enlargement must be considered. This finding alone does not always point to the enlarged right ventricle. In your differential diagnosis should be:

1. True posterior wall myocardial infarction
2. Right bundle branch block (RSR')
3. Wolff-Parkinson-White syndrome, type A

In the adult the following criteria may be found.

$Rv_1 \geq 7$ mm.
$Sv_1 \leq 2$ mm.
R/S ratio in $V_1 \geq 1$
qR pattern in V_1

Increased ventricular activation time with delayed onset of intrinsicoid deflection. (Ventricular activation time and intrinsicoid deflection are illustrated on page 362.)

Rv_5 or $Rv_6 \leq 5$ mm.
Sv_5 or $Sv_6 \geq 7$ mm.
R/S ratio in V_5 or $V_6 \leq 1$

C. Repolarization Abnormalities
(Wide QRS-T Angle and S-T Segment Abnormalities)

From Page 97 (continued) Sensitivity and Specificity

As stated in the introduction to Table 2-1, the emphasis in this course is on the concept and not on the "criteria." These criteria attempt to describe the enlarged vector of right ventricular hypertrophy (RVH). The numbers may change in the face of evolving information. The problem with the electrocardiographic recognition of right ventricular hypertrophy is that the left ventricle is dominant in the adult and even a very hypertrophied right ventricle may be overshadowed by the left ventricle. The array of criteria gives evidence that no single criterion or set of criteria have both the *sensitivity* and *specificity* desired in a diagnostic test. Most have much greater specificity than sensitivity.

Sensitivity refers to the ability of a test to yield *positive* findings among those who have the disease. It is a test that is *abnormal* when the patient *has the disease* and may be expressed (as a percentage) as follows:

$$\frac{\text{Persons with RVH and positive on the electrocardiogram}}{\text{Total number tested with RVH}} \times 100$$

Specificity refers to the ability of a test to yield a *negative* finding among those who do not have the disease. It is test that is *normal* when the patient *does not have the disease* and may be expressed (as a percentage) as follows:

$$\frac{\text{Persons without RVH and negative on the electrocardiogram}}{\text{Total number tested without RVH}} \times 100$$

From Page 97 (continued): *Ventricular Activation Time (V.A.T.) and the Intrinsicoid Deflection*[27,28]

Briefly summarized, the ventricular activation time is measured from the onset of the QRS complex to the peak of the R wave (in seconds). The peak of the R wave is also the onset of the intrinsicoid deflection. The prolonged ventricular activation time or the delayed onset of the intrinsicoid deflection has been associated with ventricular hypertrophy or ventricular conduction disturbance. The normal values are as follows:

Lead V_1—up to 0.02 sec.
Lead V_6—up to 0.04 sec.

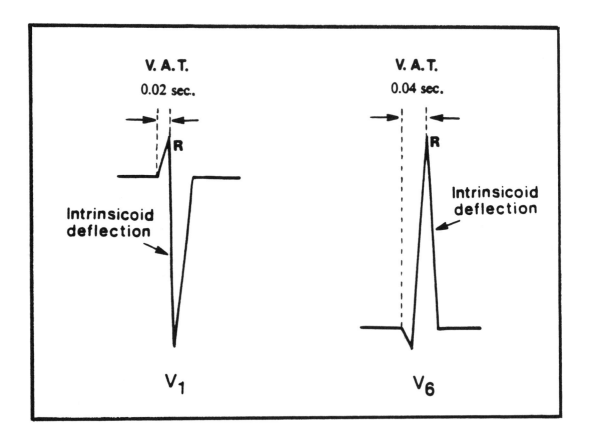

From Page 101

Although a suggested set of criteria is presented in Table 2-2, the emphasis in this course continues to be on concept. Once the basic concept of the vectorial forces of left ventricular hypertrophy is clear, the specific figures are easily understood. The values given should never be taken as absolute truths; they frequently change in the face of evolving information.

TABLE 2-2. Left Ventricular Hypertrophy

A. Increased Magnitude of the QRS Vector

Mild QRS complex prolongation may occur with increasing left ventricular hypertrophy, e.g.,
0.08-0.09-0.10-0.11 sec.

Frontal Plane Leads: I, II, III, aVR, aVL, and aVF

$R_I + S_{III}$ and/or $R_{aVL} + S_{aVF} \geq 35$ mm. (In association with left axis deviation)

$R_{aVL} \geq 12$ mm. (especially in presence of a *normally oriented* mean QRS vector)

Horizontal Plane Leads: V_1 to V_6 *(QRS magnitude criteria in an adult over the age of 30 years, of normal height and weight)*

Sv_1 or $Sv_2 + Rv_5$ or $Rv_6 \geq 35$ mm.
Sv_1 or $Sv_2 \geq 25$ mm.
Rv_5 or $Rv_6 \geq 25$ mm. (especially if $Rv_6 > Rv_5$)

B. Repolarization Abnormalities (Wide QRS-T Angle and S-T Segment Abnormalities)

C. Left Axis Deviation (LAD)

This is a conduction disturbance not necessarily associated with the hypertrophied left ventricle. Either may be found independently. It is included here because of the frequent association of LAD with left ventricular hypertrophy.

Once you are thoroughly familiar with these criteria, you will be able to scan electrocardiograms and look for left ventricular hypertrophy in the following order:

1. Increased magnitude of the mean QRS vector
2. Ventricular repolarization abnormalities
3. Left axis deviation (LAD)

From Page 101 (continued)

The many criteria recommended as evidence of left ventricular hypertrophy (LVH) attest to the fact that none have both the desired sensitivity and specificity. As in right ventricular hypertrophy, most have much greater specificity than sensitivity. Sensitivity and specificity are defined on page 361. These criteria attempt to identify the enlarged mean QRS vector of LVH. The concept of the increased vectorial magnitude will remain, although the numbers may change with new information.

Frontal plane criteria are generally less reliable than horizontal plane criteria. Furthermore, various factors, including thin chests in young patients, obesity, and bulk of intervening lung, affect the size of the QRS complex in addition to the myocardial mass. Feldman and associates recorded a 41 ± 8% increase in R wave amplitude in leads V_5 and V_6 in the change from the supine to the left lateral position.[29] The study concluded that both the size and the distance of the left ventricle to leads V_5 and V_6 are major determinants of R wave amplitude.

Additional electrocardiographic evidence of LVH is cited below under the name or names of the investigators. Owing to the large number of studies relating to all aspects of the electrocardiographic identification of LVH, these references will be restricted to QRS amplitude criteria except for the point score system of Romhilt and Estes.

Sokolow and Lyon[30]

$Sv_1 + Rv_5 > 35$ mm.
Rv_5 or $Rv_6 > 26$ mm.

Schamroth[31]

Sv_1 or $Rv_6 \geq 20$ mm.
$Sv_1 > 15$ mm. is a "pointer to potential diagnosis of LVH"

Griep,[32] and Holt and Spodick[33]

$Rv_6 > Rv_5$

Generally the R wave in lead V_5 is taller than the R wave in lead V_6. These studies indicate that if, in addition to increased QRS voltage, the R wave in lead V_6 is taller than the R wave in lead V_5, additional evidence for LVH is present.

Roberts and Day[34]
Total QRS amplitude in all 12 electrocardiographic leads > 175 mm.

From Page 101 (continued)

Casale and associates[35]

$R_{aVL} + Sv_3 > 28$ mm. in men

> 20 mm. in women

Romhilt and Estes[36]

Romhilt and Estes developed a point score system for the electrocardiographic diagnosis of left ventricular hypertrophy as follows:

		Points
1.	Amplitude Any limb lead R or S $\geq$ 20 mm. or Sv_1 or Sv_2 or $\geq$ 30 mm. or Rv_5 or $Rv_6 \geq$ 30 mm.	3
2.	ST-T abnormalities typical of LVH Without digitalis With digitalis	3
3.	Left atrial involvement Terminal negativity of Pv_1 is $\geq$ 1 mm. in depth with duration $\geq$ 0.04 sec.	3
4.	Left axis deviation $\geq -30°$ in the frontal plane.	2
5.	QRS duration $\geq$ 0.09 sec.	1
6.	Intrinsicoid deflection in V_5 or $V_6 \geq$ 0.05 sec. Maximum total 5 points signifies LVH 4 points signifies probable LVH	1 13

Biventricular Hypertrophy (RVH + LVH)

Biventricular hypertrophy is suggested by the P wave of left atrial abnormality (large left atrium as a criterion of LVH) in addition to any of the following criteria of RVH according to Murphy and associates:[37]

1. R/S ratio in lead V_5 or $V_6 \leq 1$
2. Sv_5 or $Sv_6 \geq 7$ mm. or
3. RAD of the QRS $> + 90°$.

From Page 108: Left Atrial Enlargement

Munuswamy and associates, using M-mode echocardiography, studied the sensitivity and specificity of the following six common electrocardiographic criteria for *left atrial enlargement:*[38]

1. Negative phase of Pv_1 duration > 0.04 sec.
2. Notched P wave in any standard lead with interpeak duration > 0.04 sec.
3. P-terminal force in lead V_1 > 0.04 mm./sec. (The P-terminal force in lead V_1 refers to the width (seconds) $\times$ depth (mm.) of the terminal part of the P wave)
4. Depth of negative phase of Pv_1 > 1 mm.
5. Total P wave duration in any standard lead > 0.11 sec.
6. Total P wave duration/P-R interval duration > 1.6

They found that the most *sensitive* criterion was the increased duration of the negative phase of the P wave, > 0.04 sec. in lead V_1 (83%), while the most specific was the notched P wave in any standard lead with an interpeak duration > 0.04 sec. (100%).

Josephson and associates evaluated electrocardiographic criteria for left atrial enlargement with electrophysiologic, echocardiographic, and hemodynamic correlates.[39] They concluded that the electrocardiographic manifestations of left atrial enlargement (a broad notched P wave in lead II and a deep and broad negative P wave in lead V_1) appear to represent an *interatrial conduction defect.* The term *left atrial abnormality* is commonly used.

From Page 130: *Hypokalemia*

Hypokalemia may produce striking electrocardiographic abnormalities, such as depression of the S-T segment, lowering and flattening of the T wave, and appearance of a prominent U wave. The U wave follows the T wave and has been associated with hypokalemia, although it may be found normally. The normal small U wave, when present, is seen best in the midprecordial leads. In this electrocardiogram, there appears to be a prolonged Q-T interval in lead II. The Q-T interval should be 0.28 sec., not 0.36 sec. at the rate of 125 beats per min. Lead V_2, however, reveals the hypokalemic U wave on the descending limb of the T wave. During treatment of the hypokalemia, electrocardiographic monitoring revealed a T wave that gradually became taller and a U wave that gradually disappeared. The events are graphically illustrated below. A represents the normal control with the true Q-T interval between the vertical lines. B represents lead II; the prominent U wave, if read as a T wave would lead to the wrong interpretation as a prolonged Q-T interval. C reveals both T and U waves in lead V_2.

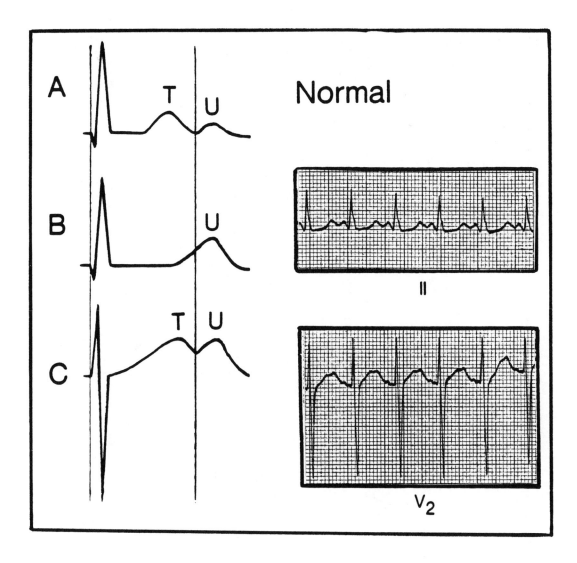

From Page 143: *Right Ventricular Infarction*

This electrocardiogram is from an elderly patient with an acute inferior (diaphragmatic) myocardial infarction. In the studies of Chou et al.[40] and Erhardt et al.[41] infarction of the right ventricle should be considered when, in addition to the findings of inferior wall infarction, there is S-T segment elevation in one (lead V_1) or more of the right precordial leads. Leads V_3R and V_4R with elevated S-T segments (arrows) reveal the involvement of the right ventricle.

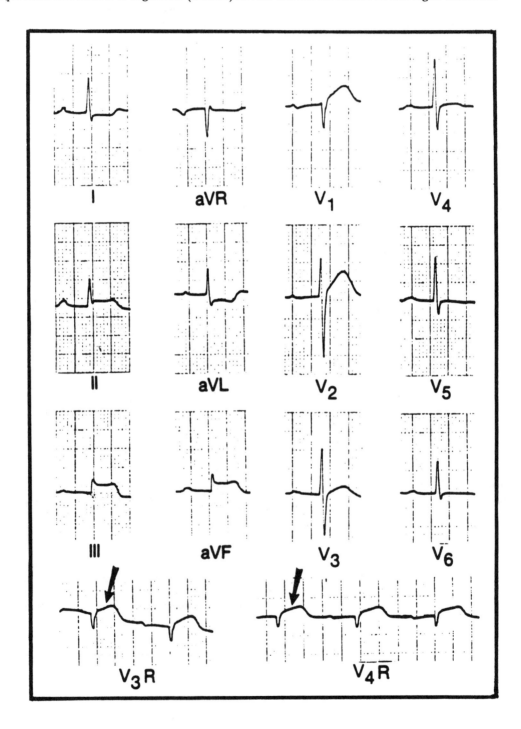

From Page 154: *Reciprocal Changes*

Note the Q waves, elevation of the S-T segments, and relatively tall T waves in leads II and III. These are the *indicative* changes in a patient with an early acute inferior (diaphragmatic) myocardial infarction. The depression of the S-T segment and inversion of the T wave in lead I, on the opposite surface of the heart, are samples of *reciprocal* changes. However, following the electrical truth learned in Chapter 1, leads I + III = lead II, the S-T segment and T wave must be negative in lead I, given the more positive S-T segment and T wave in lead III as compared with lead II. A question remains, especially in the precordial leads. Is reciprocity an electrical phenomenon only, or does it represent additional abnormalities? Numerous studies are attempting to answer this question.

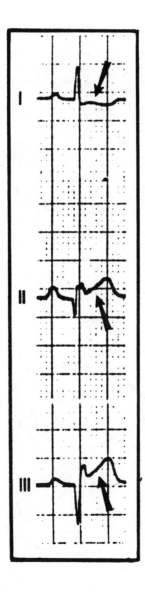

From Page 159: *Formation of the Normal Q Wave in Lead III*[42]

When the QRS vector loop, inscribed clockwise, is nearly parallel with the transition of lead III at + 30°, it may, during respiration, shift intermittently into the negative zone of lead III, inscribing a Q wave. Expiration, with the elevation of the diaphragm, tends to shift the QRS vector loop into the negative zone of lead III, inscribing a Q wave (A). Inspiration has the opposite effect, eliminating the Q wave (B).

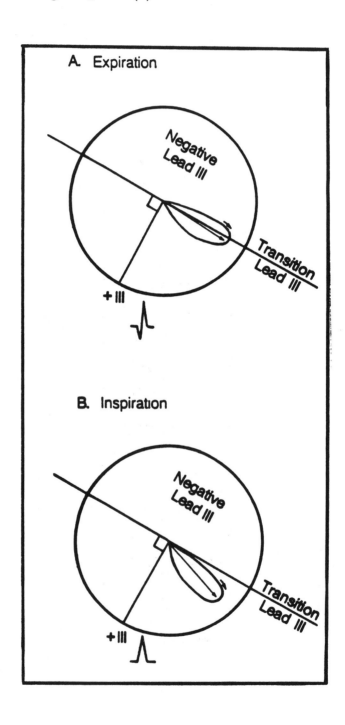

From Page 170: Mobitz Type I or Simply Type I A-V Block Ladder Diagram

A complete 4 : 3 A-V Wenckebach period is illustrated. The sinus rate is 70 per min. A-V conduction time, represented by the P-R interval, progressively increases until one beat is finally dropped. This is a typical A-V Wenckebach period. The R-R intervals decrease as the P-R intervals increase (i.e., cycle A > cycle B). The length of the pause containing the dropped beat is less than that of the two previous cycles (i.e., C < A + B); it is also less than twice the length of the previous cycle (i.e., C < 2 × B). The length of the cycle following the pause is greater than that preceding (i.e., D > B). In a 3 : 2 A-V Wenckebach period they are equal. In this case there are 4 P waves producing 3 ORS complexes, hence a 4 : 3 A-V Wenckebach period. Type I A-V block is not always associated with the Wenckebach period, but the site of block is usually the A-V node.[43] It is seldom progressive and generally reversible.

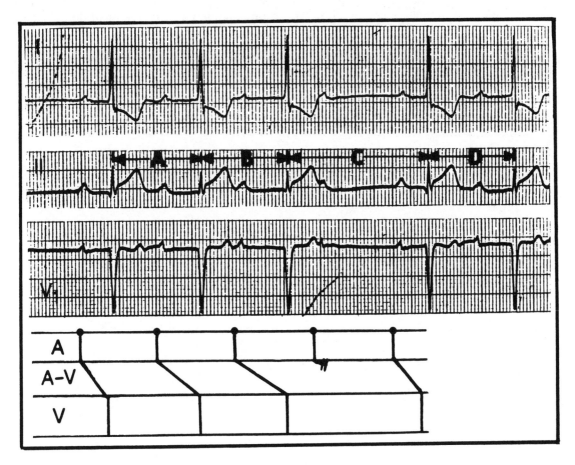

Mobitz type I A-V block.

From Page 171: Mobitz Type II or Simply Type II A-V Block Ladder Diagram

Mobitz type II A-V block represents infranodal block (His bundle block or bilateral bundle branch block). It is characterized by one or more *sudden dropped beats* with no measurable increase in the previous P-R interval. The key to the recognition of type II A-V block is the unchanging P-R interval in the consecutively conducted beats and P waves that are unexpectedly not followed by QRS complexes. Type II A-V block is a warning of future complete A-V block, as noted on page 171.

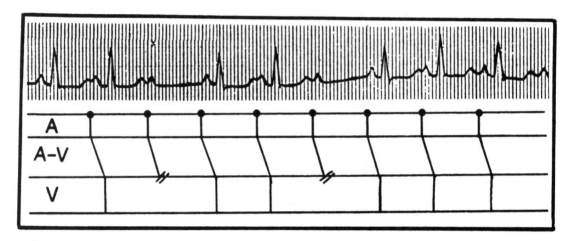

Mobitz type II A-V block. Two single dropped beats are seen. The P-R intervals of the consecutively conducted beats are unchanging.

From Page 171: Sinotrial (S-A) Wenckebach Periods

We have been studying Mobitz type I A-V block with the site of block in the A-V node. The P-P intervals are stable while there is shortening of the R-R intervals and lengthening of the P-R intervals culminating in the failure of a single beat to conduct (single dropped beat). Whereas Wenckebach conduction occurs commonly in the A-V node, the phenomenon may occur in other conducting tissue of the heart.

In *S-A Wenckebach periods,* we see the progressive shortening of the *P-P intervals* until a *P wave* is dropped. The cycle including the dropped P wave is less than two times the shortest P-P cycle. The P-R intervals are stable.

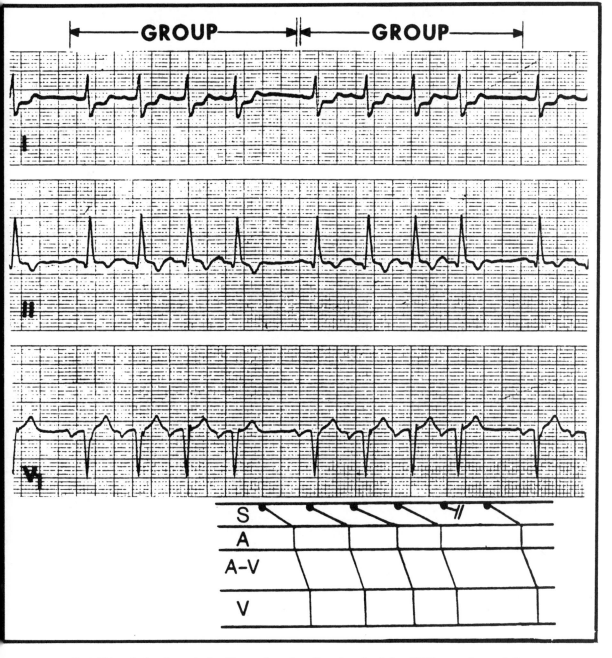

5 : 4 S-A Wenckebach periods. Group beating (brackets) of the QRS complexes follow group beating of the P waves; all P-R intervals are equal. The pause occurs when a P wave is dropped. The "S" on the ladder diagram refers to the S-A node.

From Page 173: A-V Block Versus A-V Dissociation

The terms "atrioventricular block" and "atrioventricular dissociation" are often used interchangeably. *This is not correct.* A-V block is *not* synomynous with A-V dissociation. A-V dissociation merely means that the atria and ventricles are not associated with each other. A-V block is only one category under A-V dissociation. Causes of A-V dissociation include:

1. Slowing or failure of the primary pacemaker (sinus), resulting in an escape rhythm from a lower pacemaker. This may occur in the "sick sinus" syndrome.

2. Acceleration of the subsidiary pacemaker, as may occur in accelerated junctional rhythm or ventricular tachycardia.

3. A-V block (complete: 3° degree) with slow idioventricular rhythm.

4. Combinations of 1, 2, and 3 above.

From Page 194: Critical Rate Phenomenon

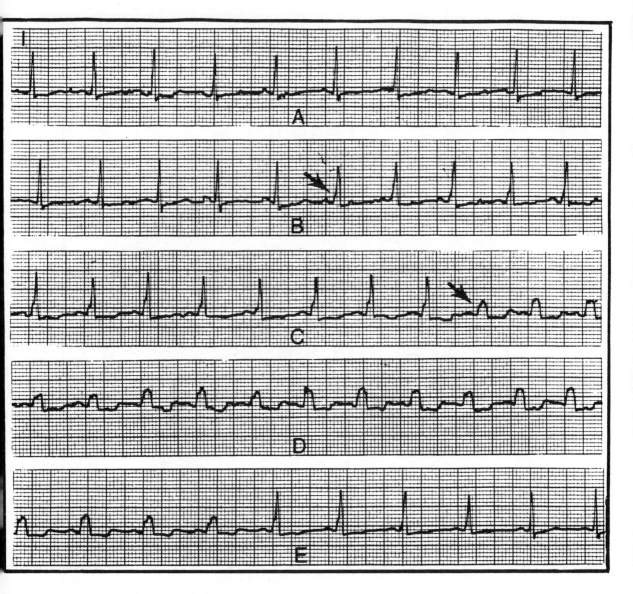

Rate dependent left bundle branch block. In panel A, at a heart rate of 90 to 93 beats per min., the QRS complex is normally narrow. As the heart rate increases to a *critical rate* of 95, the QRS complex begins to widen with the appearance of a "delta-like" wave that persists up to a rate of 100 (arrow in panel B). An electrocardiogram taken at a rate of 96 could lead to the erroneous diagnosis of the Wolff-Parkinson-White (W-P-W) syndrome. At a rate of approximately 100, the pattern of left bundle branch block is obvious (arrow in panel C) As the rate begins to slow, the left bundle branch block persists to a rate of 87, followed by the "delta-like" wave for several beats, then by the normally narrow QRS complex. Note that the *critical rate* is different as the heart rate slows (panel E). The "delta-like" wave does not represent the W-P-W syndrome, but is a step along the way toward the development of left bundle branch block at the *critical rate*. Within a few beats at *critical rates* three different conclusions may be reached:

1. Conduction with a normally narrow QRS complex
2. Erroneous diagnosis of the W-P-W syndrome
3. Left bundle branch block

Heart rate must be given due emphasis and conduction at different heart rates should be observed.

From Page 203: Modified Lead II

The single leads commonly used for the constant monitoring of arrhythmias are leads II, MCL_1, and MCL_6. Lead II is a modified lead II because the positive and negative electrodes are not placed on the respective extremities, but on the chest as illustrated below. MCL_1 and MCL_6 are illustrated on the following page.

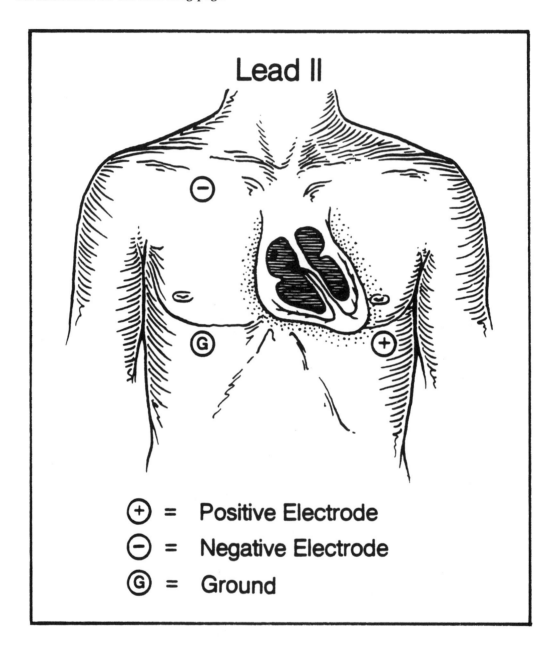

Lead II

$\oplus$ = Positive Electrode
$\ominus$ = Negative Electrode
G = Ground

From Page 203 (continued): Leads MCL$_1$ and MCL$_6$

MCL$_1$ and MCL$_6$ are also modified leads because the negative electrode is near the left shoulder and not on the left arm (in the "unmodified" CL lead the negative electrode is placed on the left arm and the positive on the chest as illustrated below).

M = modified
C = chest (positive electrode)
L = left arm (negative electrode)

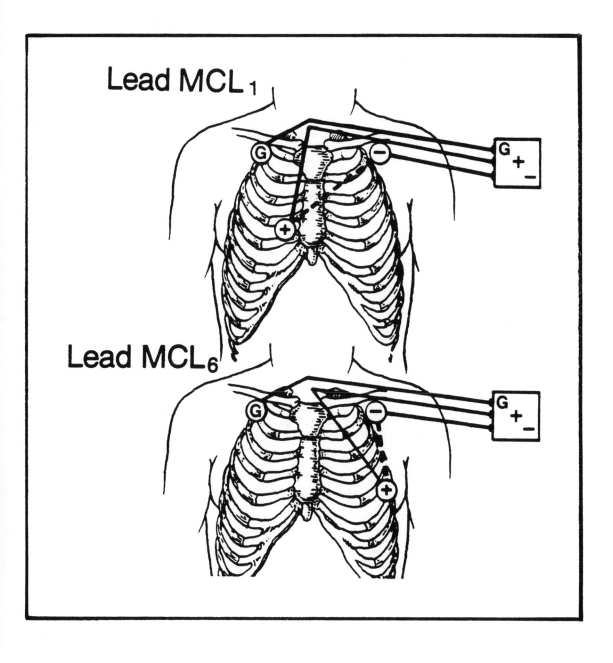

From Page 209: Ladder Diagram of Sinus Arrhythmia

Complete the ladder diagram of this example of sinus arrhythmia.

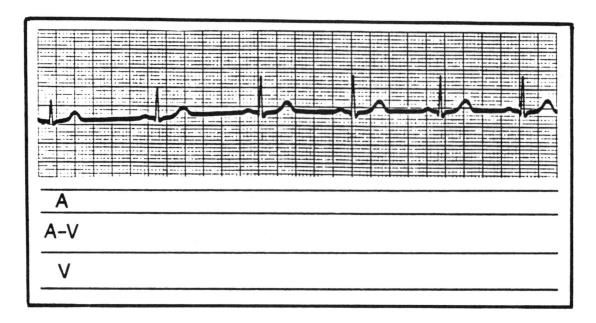

Solution:

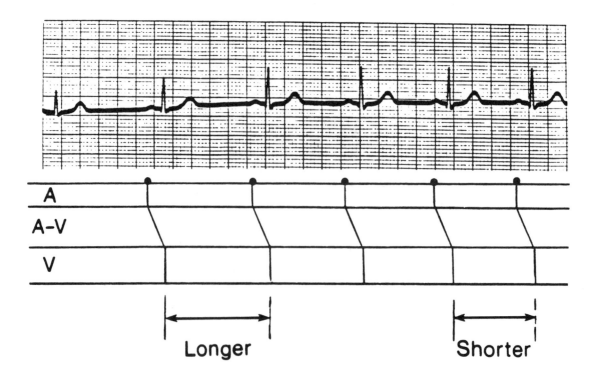

From Page 210: S-A Block

The electrocardiographic tracings are from the same patient as on page 210. The upper panel could be mistaken for sinus bradycardia. The middle and lower panels prove the rhythm to be intermittent 2 : 1 S-A block with sudden doubling of the P-P intervals.

Compare this electrocardiogram with type I A-V block (page 371), type II A-V block (page 372), and the electrocardiogram on page 373 with S-A Wenckebach periods.

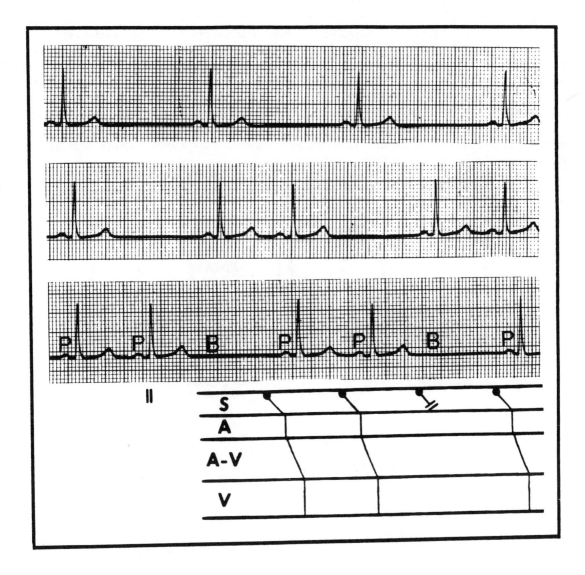

From Page 215: Reentry and Enhanced Automaticity

It is important to understand the concept of reentry because it is the mechanism of most supraventricular and many ventricular tachycardias. A in the schematic represents a normal transmission of an impulse, coming down two parallel pathways with no interruption. To have a reentrant (reciprocal) mechanism there must be two conduction pathways differering in refractoriness and conduction velocity, B and C, representing different stages in the same reentry circuit in the A-V node. The circuit consists of a slow and a fast pathway with a final common pathway at either end. The slow pathway has slow conduction, but a relatively short antegrade refractory period. The fast pathway has more rapid antegrade conduction and a relatively short retrograde (backward) refractory period. Under certain conditions, an antegrade impulse may be blocked in the fast pathway while conducting slowly down the slow pathway. Given a critical degree of slowing, an impulse may arrive at the lower reaches of the A-V node via the slow pathway and find the fast pathway already recovered and able to conduct in the retrograde direction. The impulse then travels up the fast pathway to the upper reaches of the A-V node, from where it may (1) stimulate the atrium in retrograde fashion, and/or (2) find the slow pathway able to conduct in the antegrade direction, thus beginning another reentry loop, leading to a tachycardia. If one loop is made by the impulse, an extrasystole results.

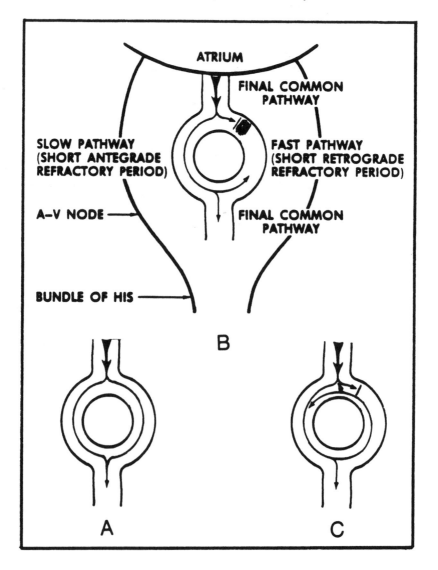

Model for A-V nodal reentry.[44]

From Page 215 (continued)

The A-V node was used as an example of a reentry circuit. A reentry circuit may occur in other sites in the heart such as the Purkinje fiber system. Reentry involving the A-V node and bundle of Kent is illustrated below.

Tachycardias may result from reentry as previously described or from a rapidly firing ectopic focus (enhanced automaticity). Ectopic beats are beats arising in any focus other than the S-A node. Automaticity is a property of pacemaking cells which form impulses spontaneously.

Some examples of reentrant (reciprocating) tachycardias are paroxysmal supraventricular tachycardia, ventricular tachycardia, pre-excitation (L-G-L and W-P-W) tachycardia and coupled premature beats. Examples of automatic tachycardias include atrial tachycardia with block and nonparoxysmal junctional tachycardia, both due to digitalis toxicity, ectopic atrial tachycardia, multifocal atrial tachycardia, and idioventricular rhythm.

In the reentrant or reciprocating supraventricular tachycardia illustrated below, a reentry loop became established within the A-V node, a common site.

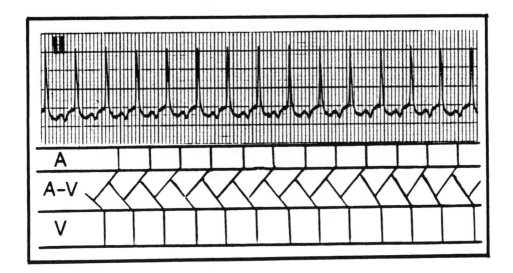

Reentrant (reciprocating) supraventricular tachycardia.

From Page 215 (continued)

The common reentrant circuit in W-P-W tachycardias involves antegrade conduction in the A-V node and retrograde conduction through the bundle of Kent, producing a normal narrow QRS complex. Much less common is antegrade conduction through the bundle of Kent with retrograde conduction through the A-V node, producing a wide, bizarre QRS complex.

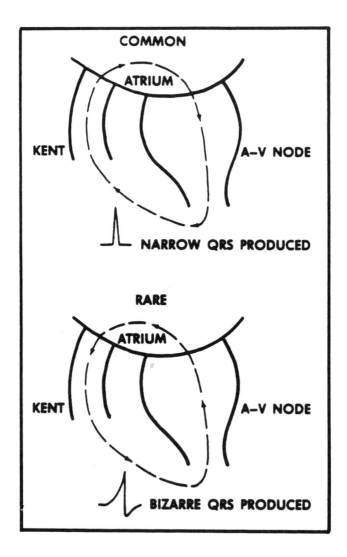

Reentry invoking the A-V node and bundle of Kent.[45]

From Page 220: Junctional Rhythm P Waves

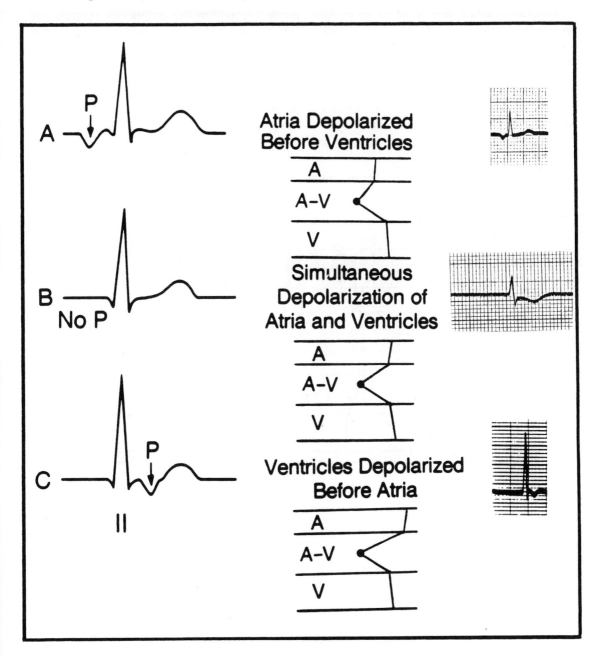

Ladder diagrams of the three examples presented on page 220.

From Page 233: Concealed Conduction

Concealed conduction refers to an impulse, conducted within the conduction system, not visible (concealed) on the electrocardiogram, which influences the subsequent cycle. Using the example of the partial compensatory pause, note that the P-R interval of the fourth cycle is greater than the P-R intervals of cycles 1, 2 and 5. The PVC (4) penetrated the A-V junction sufficiently so that when the next sinus P wave came at the regular P-P interval, it encountered the A-V junction partially refractory resulting in delayed conduction in the A-V junction and prolonged P-R interval. The retrograde penetration of the A-V junction is an example of *concealed conduction* within the A-V junction (C on the ladder diagram) because it cannot be seen on the electrocardiogram but its effect is seen on the next cycle.

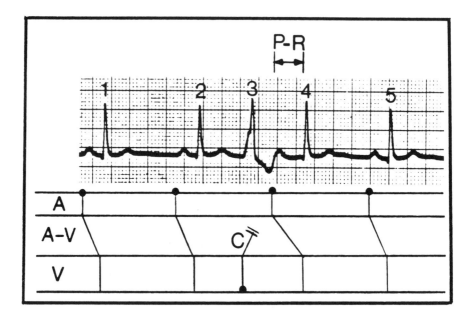

Concealed conduction.

From Page 238: "Rule of Bigeminy"

Langendorf, Pick, and Winternitz, in proposing the "rule of bigeminy," stated that "lengthening of the ventricular cycle favors the appearance of ventricular premature systoles. . . .once ventricular bigeminy is initiated. . ., it tends to persist because of the long pause which follows each premature systole. . . ."[46]

This was illustrated on page 238 and is reproduced here.

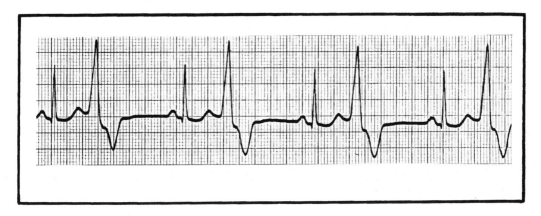

Bigeminy.

From Page 240: Fusion

A fusion beat occurs when more than one impulse conducts through the same myocardial area at approximately the same time, fusing into one beat. Fusion beats may occur in the ventricles or atria. The fusion beat (F below) is evident when the supraventricular impulse (in this case the sinus impulse) enters the ventricles at approximately the same time as an ectopic ventricular impulse fusing into one beat. Note that the P-R interval preceding the fusion beat is almost identical to the other P-R intervals. The underlying rhythm is sinus with 2 : 1 A-V block.

When the QRS complexes are wide, the presence of fusion beats favors ventricular ectopy rather than aberrant ventricular conduction (pages 391 and 392). Fusion beats may be seen with PVCs, as in this electrocardiogram, during ventricular arrhythmias (accelerated idioventricular rhythm and ventricular tachycardia), ventricular pacing and ventricular parasystole. Atrial fusion may occur with simultaneous impulses from the S-A node and A-V junction depolarizing the atria.

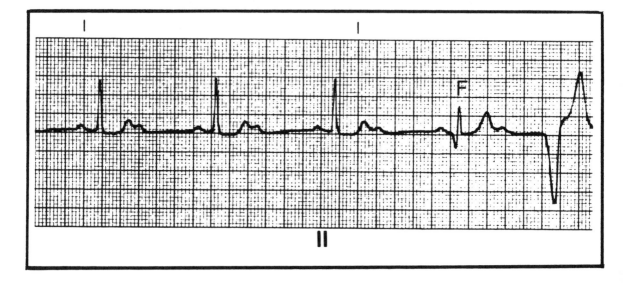

Fusion. The first of the two PVCs is in fusion (F). The underlying rhythm is sinus with 2 : 1 A-V block.

From Page 240: Fusion (continued)

Dressler and Roesler stressed the contribution of fusion beats in the recognition of ventricular tachycardia.[47] They presented cases of ventricular tachycardia "which show variations of the ventricular complexes transitional in shape to sinoauricular beats. The variations are caused by the transmission of atrial excitations to the ventricles, which mostly results in ventricular fusion beats." These fusion beats are often called Dressler beats.

The electrocardiogram illustrates ventricular tachycardia with fusion (F) beats.

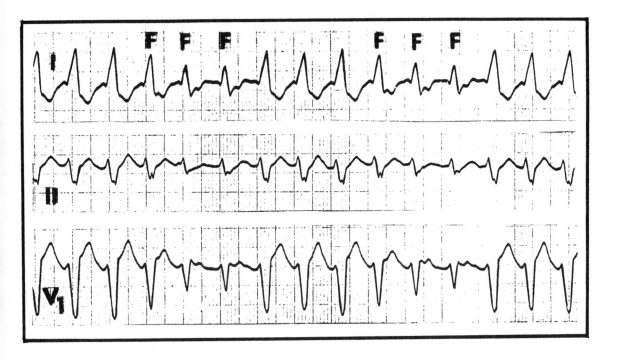

Fusion beats in ventricular tachycardia.

From Page 240 (continued): Parasystole

Under normal circumstances, the many latent pacemakers of the heart are continually pene-trated and reset by the impulses arising in the S-A node. In this manner, they remain suppressed by the usually faster sinus. When a latent pacemaker acquires a protective shell of refractory tissue that prevents its penetration by the sinus, it may then reach threshold and discharge. Such a protected latent pacemaker is termed a parasystole, and may be located in the atria, junction, or ventricles. Upon firing, a parasystolic focus may find its impulse blocked either because the surrounding tissue has been rendered refractory by a sinus beat that it follows too closely, or because the immediately surrounding tissue is refractory because of intrinsic reasons.

On the electrocardiogram, a parasystole is recognized when a series of atrial, junctional, or ventricular extrasystoles are found to be related to each other, rather than either fixed-coupled to the dominant rhythm or randomly occurring. The interectopic intervals may be constant or varying. If varying, either the longer intervals are multiples of the shorter intervals, or all the intervals are multiples of some shorter interval not present. Fusion beats of the ectopic beats and normally conducted beats are common and must be counted when determining the interectopic intervals.

Ventricular parasystole is illustrated in this electrocardiogram. The diagnostic features are
1. Nonfixed coupling between the normally conducted beats and the PVCs.
2. Fusion (F) of a ventricular beat and a normally conducted beat.
3. Regular interectopic and a multiple of the basic interectopic interval.

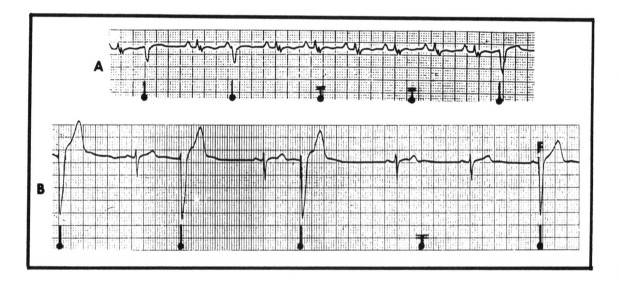

Ventricular parasystole. Unifocal nonfixed-coupled PVCs are present. A. The long PVC cycle is equal to three short cycles. B. One fusion beat (F) is present. The long PVC cycle is equal to two short cycles. (The basic parasytolic cycle length varies slightly.)

From Page 240: Parasystole (continued)

In junctional parasystole (below) nonfixed-coupled premature junctional contractions (PJCs) are present. All junctional cycles are multiples of a basic cycle.

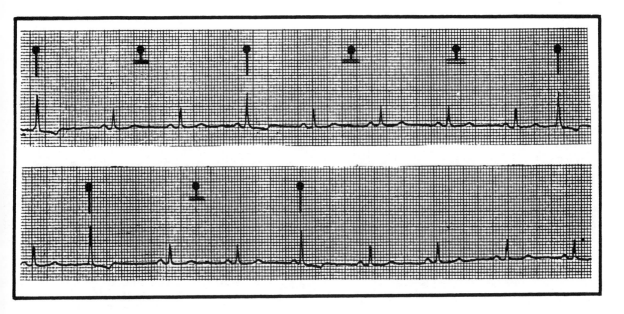

Junctional parasystole.

From Page 243: Wide QRS Complex

The width of the QRS complex is helpful in the distinction between a supraventricular and a ventricular rhythm.

1. A normally narrow (up to 0.1 sec.) QRS complex indicates a supraventricular rhythm (sinus, atrial, or junctional).
2. A ventricular rhythm has an abnormally wide QRS complex (usually 0.12 sec. or wider).

There is an exception, however. In the illustrations below (A and B), we have all the requirements of normal sinus rhythm except the QRS complex is wide (greater than 0.1 sec). The rhythms are *supraventricular with a P wave preceding each QRS complex at a fixed P-R interval.* Because there is an intraventricular conduction disturbance, left bundle branch block (LBBB) in A and right bundle branch block (RBBB) in B, with delayed ventricular depolarization, there is a *wide* QRS complex.

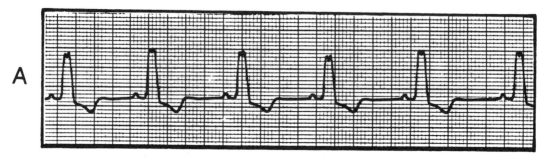

Left bundle branch block (LBBB).

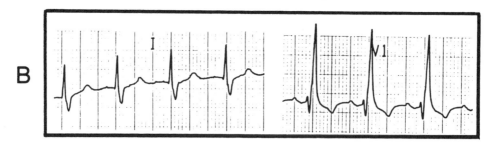

Right bundle branch block (RBBB).

These supraventricular rhythms with wide QRS complexes are easily recognizable because the P waves preceding each QRS complex are clearly seen. During tachycardia, when the P waves may not be obvious, the distinction between a supraventricular rhythm and a ventricular rhythm may not be as evident.

It is important to recognize LBBB and RBBB in order to understand the supraventricular rhythms with a wide QRS complex and the subject of aberrant ventricular conduction, which will be studied shortly.

From Page 243 (continued): Aberrant Ventricular Conduction or Aberrancy Including the Ashman Phenomenon

Aberrant ventricular conduction, or aberrancy, refers to abnormal ventricular depolarization following conduction of a supraventricular impulse. This occurs when a supraventricular impulse arrives while the ventricles are still partially refractory. In the example below, a premature supraventricular impulse found the right bundle branch refractory, hence the wide QRS complex of right bundle branch block (arrow) representing aberrant ventricular conduction. The wide QRS complex with the pattern of either RBBB or LBBB and preceding associated atrial activity indicates that the origin of the impulse is supraventricular.

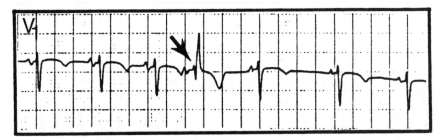

Aberrant ventricular conduction.

The refractory period of the conduction system adjusts to the heart rate, shortening with increasing heart rates (shorter cycles) and lengthening with lower heart rates (longer cycles). During the long cycle the refractory period lengthens and when a short cycle follows, the ventricular conduction system is still partially refractory, leading to aberrant ventricular conduction. This was described by Gouaux and Ashman in patients with atrial fibrillation and is known as the Ashman phenomenon.[48] In the electrocardiogram below note the aberrant ventricular conduction in a patient in atrial fibrillation with long (A)-short (B) cycles. Single aberrant beats or the first aberrant beat of each multiple terminates a "long-short" sequence.

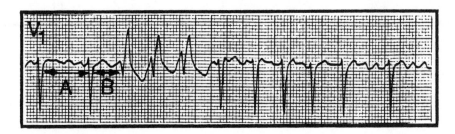

Ashman phenomenon.

From page 243 (continued)

In differentiating aberrant ventricular conduction with a supraventricular pacemaker from ventricular ectopic beats, atrial activity and a RBBB or LBBB pattern point toward aberrant ventricular conduction. The availability of a baseline electrocardiogram with a bundle branch block pattern helps us, especially during a tachycardia, in determining the origin of the impulse. Below is the electrocardiogram of a patient with a wide QRS tachycardia (A), whose baseline electrocardiogram revealed the same LBBB pattern (B). The diagnosis of supraventricular tachycardia can then be made with security.

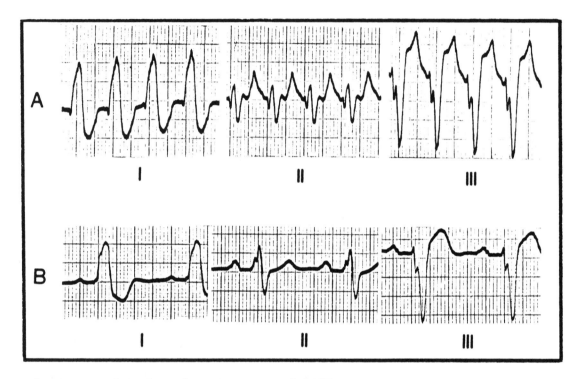

Supraventricular tachycardia in a patient with LBBB.

From Page 243 (continued): His Bundle Studies

All the heartbeat disorders have been under intensive investigation. Proliferation of coronary care units has given great impetus to this study; many arrhythmias arising in the patient with a myocardial infarction may be stopped or prevented entirely. Methods have been developed that help in the interpretation of arrhythmias and facilitate understanding of the underlying electrophysiologic principles. Among these has been the technique of His bundle recording for clinical use, which was developed in our laboratory and represents one of the great advances in cardiology.[49] The His bundle study is a technique where an electrode catheter is placed near the tricuspid valve via the femoral vein or an arm vein and recordings are made from the area of the His bundle. We see a sharp deflection, labeled H in the illustration below, between the atrial and ventricular deflections. His bundle recordings have terminated the "silence" of the P-R segment.

In the illustration from above down are seen standard leads I, II, and III, in addition to recordings from within the heart. HBE is the His bundle electrogram; A, atrial deflection; H, His deflection; V, ventricular deflection. The three ventricular deflections are labeled 1, 2, and 3. Ventricular complexes 1 and 2 are preceded by an atrial deflection (a), lining up with the P wave on the clinical electrocardiogram, and a His deflection (H), representing normal A-V conduction. Complex 3, the premature beat, is not preceded by a P wave, only by a His deflection. It is a junctional or His bundle premature beat. If a His deflection precedes the QRS complex it is likely to be a *supraventricular* beat. Ventricular beats would not be preceded by His deflections at a fixed interval. The third A, following the premature contraction, is of sinus origin, which cannot conduct to the ventricles because the ventricular conduction system is in a refractory state because of the premature contraction.

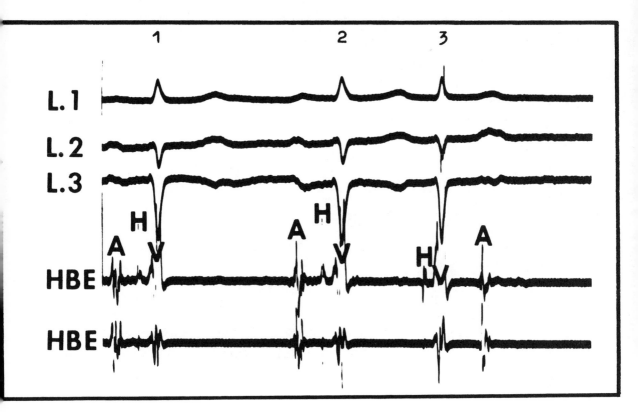

His bundle study.

From Page 243: Wolff-Parkinson-White (W-P-W) and
Lown-Ganong-Levine (L-G-L) Syndromes (Pre-excitation)

WOLFF-PARKINSON-WHITE (W-P-W) SYNDROME

Another example of a wide QRS complex with a supraventricular pacemaker is the W-P-W syndrome. In 1930 Louis Wolff, John Parkinson, and Paul Dudley White published their classic study of 11 cases entitled: "Bundle branch block with short P-R interval in healthy young people prone to paroxysmal tachycardia.[50] This is known universally as the Wolff-Parkinson-White or W-P-W syndrome. It does not represent bundle branch block as was once thought. Wolff, in a later paper, enumerated the various names given to this syndrome as the Wolff-Parkinson-White (W-P-W) syndrome, anomalous atrioventricular excitation, the syndrome of the short P-R interval with abnormal QRS complexes and paroxysmal tachycardia, pre-excitation, and the bundle of Kent syndrome.[51] The electrocardiographic pattern is characterized by a:

1. Short P-R interval (0.12 sec. or less)
2. Prolonged QRS interval (greater than 0.1 sec)
3. Slurring of the upstroke by a *delta* wave

The mechanism responsible for this syndrome is illustrated below. There is an accessory atrioventricular pathway, the bundle of Kent, in addition to the A-V node. Conduction from the atria to the ventricles through the accessory pathway occurs before the normal conduction through the A-V node resulting in pre-excitation of the ventricles. Pre-excitation refers to the earlier

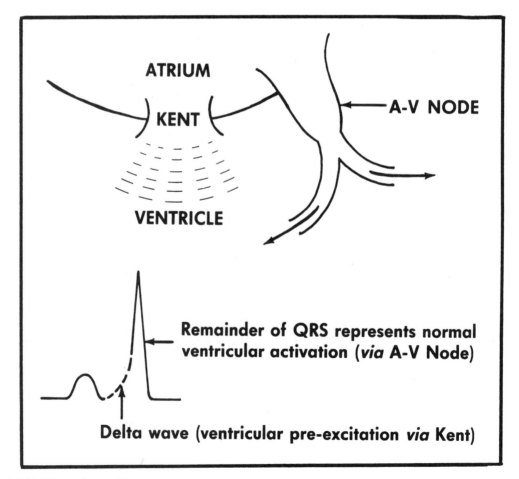

W-P-W syndrome.[52]

W-P-W SYNDROME (Continued)

activation of the ventricles than would normally be expected. Conduction through the accessory pathway bypasses the A-V node and its normal delay. Because this pre-excitation results in asynchronous activation of the ventricles, a wide and abnormal appearing QRS deflection is inscribed. Usually, before completion of this deflection, the remainder of ventricular activation is through the normal conduction system. The resulting QRS complex, therefore, begins with a slurred upstroke known as the *delta* wave (conduction through the bundle of Kent).

The important features of the Wolff-Parkinson-White syndrome include the following:

1. The association of the W-P-W syndrome with supraventricular tachycardis—namely reentrant (reciprocating) supraventricular tachycardia, atrial fibrillation, and atrial flutter. Review the mechanism of reentry and the pathways of reentry in the W-P-W syndrome on pages 380 to 382.
2. The alternation of normal conduction with the W-P-W syndrome is frequent and can make the search for the cause of a supraventricular tachycardia difficult. The electrocardiogram below illustrates delta waves, which were seen only intermittently.

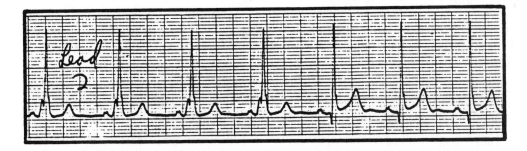

Intermittent delta waves in the W-P-W syndrome.

From Page 243 (continued):

LOWN-GANONG-LEVINE (L-G-L) SYNDROME

Lown, Ganong, and Levine described the syndrome of the short P-R interval (less than 0.12 sec.), *normal* QRS complex, and paroxysmal rapid heart action.[53] Caracta and associates studied 18 patients with a short P-R interval (<0.12 sec.) and normal QRS complex:[54] Eight had a history of supraventricular tachycardia. Among the possible explanations for the short P-R interval were the following:

1. Total or partial bypass of the A-V node
2. An anatomically small A-V node
3. Short or rapidly conducting intranodal pathway

Benditt and associates demonstrated that A-V nodal refractory periods were shorter and enhanced A-V conduction more frequent in L-G-L patients compared with normal controls.[55] Josephson and Kastor studied the mechanism of the abbreviated A-V nodal conduction time and paroxysmal supraventricular tachycardia in six patients with the L-G-L syndrome.[56] Their findings include dual A-V nodal pathways and suggested that preferential rapidly conducting A-V nodal fibers and intranodal reentry are the responsible mechanisms in these patients with the L-G-L syndrome and reciprocating tachycardia.

Of historical interest, Katz and Pick called this rhythm the *coronary nodal rhythm,* stating that "it is diagnosed when, with the P-R interval between 0.02 and 0.10 second, the P waves in leads I and II are upright. Usually the P-R interval is nearer 0.10 second."[57]

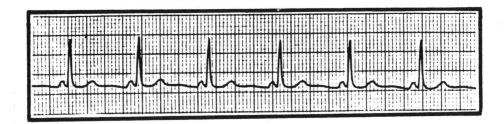

L-G-L syndrome.

REFERENCES

1. Beckwith, J.: Grant's Clinical Electrocardiography, 2nd Ed. New York, McGraw-Hill, 1970.
2. Stein, E.: Clinical Electrocardiography: A Self-Study Course. Philadelphia, Lea & Febiger, 1987.
3. Stein, E.: Electrocardiographic Interpretation: A Self-Study Approach to Clinical Electrocardiography. Philadelphia, Lea & Febiger, 1991.
4. Fox, W., and Stein, E.: Cardiac Rhythm Disturbances: A Step-by-Step Approach. Philadelphia, Lea & Febiger, 1983.
5. Wasserburger, R. H.: Observations on the "juvenile pattern" of adult Negro males. Am. J. Med., *18:* 428, 1955.
6. Reiley, M. A., et al.: Racial and sexual differences in the standard electrocardiogram of black vs white adolescents. Chest, *75:* 474, 1979.
7. Kambara, H., and Phillips, J.: Long-term evaluation of early repolarization syndrome (normal variant RS-T segment elevation). Am. J. Cardiol., *38:* 157, 1976.
8. Mirvis, D.: Evaluation of normal variations in S-T segment patterns by body surface isopotential mapping: S-T segment elevation in absence of heart disease. Am. J. Cardiol., *50:* 122, 1982.
9. Spodick, D. H.: Differential characteristics of the electrocardiogram in early repolarization and acute pericarditis. N. Engl. J. Med., *295:* 523, 1976.
10. Spodick, D. H.: Pathogenesis and clinical correlations of the electrocardiographic abnormalities of pericardial disease. Cardiovasc. Clin., *8:* 201, 1977.
11. Ginzton, L. E., and Laks, M. M.: The differential diagnosis of acute pericarditis from the normal variant: new electrocardiographic criteria. Circulation, *65:* 1004, 1982.
12. Amsterdam, E. A., et al.: Toward improved interpretation of the exercise test. Cardiology, *66:* 236, 1980.
13. Prinzmetal, M., et al.: Angina pectoris. I. A variant form of angina pectoris. Am. J. Med., *27:* 375, 1959.
14. Prinzmetal, M., et al.: Variant form of angina pectoris, previously undelineated syndrome. JAMA, *174:* 1794, 1960.
15. Palmer, J. H.: Isolated U wave negativity. Circulation, *7:* 205, 1953.
16. Kishida, H., et al.: Negative U wave: a highly specific but poorly understood sign of heart disease. Am. J. Cardiol., *49:* 2030, 1982.
17. Barold, S. S.: Modern Cardiac Pacing. Mt. Kisco, NY, Futura, 1985.
18. Barold, S. S.: New Perspectives in Cardiac Pacing. Mt. Kisco, NY, Futura, 1988.
19. Furman, S. et al.: A Practice of Cardiac Pacing. Mt. Kisco, NY, Futura, 1986.
20. Gillette, P. C., and Griffin, J. C.: Practical Cardiac Pacing. Baltimore, Williams & Wilkins, 1986.
21. Horan, L., et al.: The significance of diagnostic Q waves in the presence of bundle branch block. Chest, *58:* 214, 1970.
22. Havelda, C. J., et al.: The pathologic correlates of the electrocardiogram: complete left bundle branch block. Circulation, *65:* 445, 1982.
23. Park, M. K. and Guntheroth, W. G.: How to Read Pediatric ECGs. Chicago, Year Book, 1981.
24. Schamroth, L.: The 12 Lead Electrocardiogram. Oxford, Blackwell Scientific Publications, 1989, p. 11.
25. Marriott, H. J. L.: Practical Electrocardiography, 8th Ed. Baltimore, Williams & Wilkins, 1988, p. 44.
26. Nadas, A. S., and Fyler, D. C.: Pediatric Cardiology, 3rd Ed. Philadelphia, W. B. Saunders, 1972.
27. Schamroth, L: The 12 Lead Electrocardiogram. Oxford, Blackwell Scientific Publications, 1989, p. 5.
28. Marriott, H. J. L.: Practical Electrocardiography, 8th Ed. Baltimore, Williams & Wilkins, 1988, p. 41.

29. Feldman, T., et al.: Relation of electrocardiographic R-wave amplitude to changes in left ventricular chamber size and position in normal subjects. Am. J. Cardiol., *55:* 1168, 1985.

30. Sokolow, M., and Lyon, T. P.: The ventricular complex in left ventricular hypertrophy as obtained by unipolar precordial and limb leads. Am. Heart J., *37:* 161, 1949.

31. Schamroth, L.: The 12 Lead Electrocardiogram. Oxford, Blackwell Scientific Publications, 1989, p. 34.

32. Griep, A. H.: Pitfalls in electrocardiographic diagnosis of left ventricular hypertrophy: a correlative study of 200 autopsied patients. Circulation, *20:* 30, 1959.

33. Holt, D. H., and Spodick, D. H.: The Rv_6:Rv_5 voltage ratio in left ventricular hypertrophy. Am. Heart J., *63:* 65, 1962.

34. Roberts, W. C., and Day, P. J.: Electrocardiographic observations in clinically isolated, pure, chronic severe aortic regurgitation: analysis of 30 necropsy patients aged 19 to 65 years. Am. J. Cardiol., *55:* 431, 1985.

35. Casale, P. N., et al.: Improved sex-specific criteria of left ventricular hypertrophy for clinical and computer interpretation of electrocardiograms: validation with autopsy findings. Circulation, *75:* 565, 1987.

36. Romhilt, D. W., and Estes, E. H.: A point-score system for the ECG diagnosis of left ventricular hypertrophy. Am. Heart J., *6:* 752, 1968.

37. Murphy, M. L., et al.: Reevaluation of electrocardiographic criteria for left, right and combined cardiac ventricular hypertrophy. Am. J. Cardiol., *53:* 1140, 1984.

38. Munuswamy, K., et al.: Sensitivity and specificity of commonly used electrocardiographic criteria for left atrial enlargement determined by M-mode echocardiography. Am. J. Cardiol., *53:* 829, 1984.

39. Josephson, M. E., et al.: Electrocardiographic left atrial enlargement: electrophysiologic, echocardiographic and hemodynamic correlates. Am. J. Cardiol., *39:* 967, 1977.

40. Chou, T.-C., et al.: Electrocardiographic diagnosis of right ventricular infarction. Am. J. Med., *70:* 1175, 1981.

41. Erhardt, L. R., et al.: Single right-sided precordial lead in the diagnosis of right ventricular involvement in inferior myocardial infarction. Am. Heart J., *91:* 571, 1976.

42. Schamroth, L.: The 12 Lead Electrocardiogram. Oxford, Blackwell Scientific Publications, 1989, p. 158.

43. Marriott, H. J. L.: Practical Electrocardiography. 8th Ed. Baltimore, Williams & Wilkins, 1988. p. 386.

44. Fox, W., and Stein, E.: Cardiac Rhythm Disturbances: A Step-by-Step Approach. Philadelphia, Lea & Febiger, 1983, p. 12.

45. Fox, W., and Stein, E.: Cardiac Rhythm Disturbances: A Step-by-Step Approach. Philadelphia, Lea & Febiger, 1983, p. 13.

46. Langendorf, R., et al.: Mechanisms of intermittent ventricular bigeminy; I. Appearance of ectopic beats dependent upon the length of the ventricular cycle, the "rule of bigeminy." Circulation, *11:* 442, 1955.

47. Dressler, W., and Roesler, H.: The occurrence in paroxysmal tachycardia of ventricular complexes transitional in shape to sinoauricular beats. Am. Heart J., *44:* 485, 1952.

48. Gouaux, J. L., and Ashman, R.: Auricular fibrillation with aberration simulating ventricular paroxysmal tachycardia. Am. Heart J., *34:* 366, 1947.

49. Scherlag, B. J., et al.: Catheter technique for recording His bundle activity in man. Circulation, *39:* 13, 1969.

50. Wolff, L., Parkinson, J., and White, P. D.: Bundle branch block with short P-R interval in healthy young people prone to paroxysmal tachycardia. Am. Heart J., *5:* 685, 1930.

51. Wolff, L.: Syndrome of short P-R interval with abnormal QRS complexes and paroxysmal tachycardia (Wolff-Parkinson-White syndrome). Circulation, *10:* 282, 1954.

52. Fox, W., and Stein, E.: Cardiac Rhythm Disturbances: A Step-by-Step Approach. Philadelphia, Lea & Febiger, 1983, p. 162.

53. Lown, B., Ganong, W. R., and Levine, S. A.: The syndrome of short P-R interval, normal QRS complex and paroxysmal rapid heart action. Circulation, *5:* 693, 1952.

54. Caracta, A. R., et al.: Electrophysiologic studies in the syndrome of short P-R interval, normal QRS complex. Am. J. Cardiol., *31:* 245, 1973.
55. Benditt, D. G., et al.: Characteristics of atrioventricular conduction and the spectrum of arrhythmias in Lown-Ganong-Levine syndrome. Circulation, *57:* 454, 1978.
56. Josephson, M. E., and Kastor, J. A.: Supraventricular tachycardia in Lown-Ganong-Levine syndrome: atrionodal versus intranodal reentry. Am. J. Cardiol., *40:* 521, 1977.
57. Katz, L. N., and Pick, A.: Clinical Electrocardiography: The Arrhythmias. Philadelphia, Lea & Febiger, 1956, p. 102.

Index